W9-BLY-412

To access your Student Resources, visit the web address below:

http://evolve.elsevier.com/Chabner/Short

Evolve Student Learning Resources for *Chabner: Medical Terminology A Short Course, 4th edition* offers the following features:

- ## Chapter Quizzes
  Provides additional self-testing of medical terms with instant feedback.

- ## Body Spectrum Electronic Anatomy Coloring Book
  Provides 80 anatomy illustrations that can be colored online or printed out for coloring and study offline. Choose from a varied color palette and learn anatomy in this fun, interactive format. Test your knowledge by completing quizzes after each part is colored.

- ## Commonly Used Medical Word Parts
  Provides a quick reference of commonly used medical word parts.

- ## English-Spanish Glossary
  A glossary of medical terms with the Spanish translations.

Davi-Ellen Chabner, BA, MAT

Medical Terminology

4th edition

A Short Course

ELSEVIER
SAUNDERS

ELSEVIER
SAUNDERS

11830 Westline Industrial Drive
St. Louis, Missouri 63146

MEDICAL TERMINOLOGY: A SHORT COURSE, Fourth Edition
Copyright © 2005, 2003, 1999, 1991 by Elsevier Inc.

ISBN-13: 978–1–4160–0165–2
ISBN-10: 1–4160–0165–4

Acquisitions Editor: Jeanne Wilke
Developmental Editor: Becky Swisher
Publishing Services Manager: Patricia Tannian
Senior Project Manager: Anne Altepeter
Senior Book Designer: Ellen Zanolle

Printed in China

Last digit is the print number: 9 8 7 6 5 4 3 2

Reviewers

Angela D. Anderson, MA, RT (R) (CT) (QM)
Radiography Program Director
Prince George's Community College
Largo, Maryland

G. Audrey Beati, RN, BSN
Health/Medical Instructor
Greater Lowell Technical High School
Tyngsboro, Massachusetts

Jennifer M. Evans
Coordinator for Medical Office CIST
    and Instructor
South Seattle Community College
Seattle, Washington

Marie A. Fenske, EdD, RRT
Faculty, Coordinator of Healthcare
    Core
GateWay Community College
Phoenix, Arizona

Cindy Anne Henley, RN, MSN, GNP
John A. Logan College
Carterville, Illinois

Diane Michele Langone, LPN, RHIA
Medical Terminology Course
    Instructor
Mohawk Valley Community College
Utica, New York
Teaching Assistant for Nursing
    Theory and Procedures
Madison/Oneida BOCES
Verona, New York

Patricia Kaye Leary
Allied Health Instructor
Mecosta Osceola Career Center
Ferris State University
Big Rapids, Michigan

Patricia Roberto, MA, BVE
Professor
Cerritos College
Norwalk, California
Instructor
Computer Training Center
ABC Adult School
Cerritos, California

To my grandchildren

For the great happiness they give me

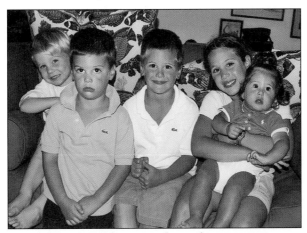

Ben, Gus, Solomon, Bebe, and Louisa Rose

and

To Eli (1991-2004)

For years of devotion, companionship, and love

Preface

I am pleased to present the fourth edition of *Medical Terminology: A Short Course*. Its upbeat, dynamic appearance will draw you into the exciting world of medical terminology. This edition contains **new images** of anatomical and pathological terminology. Features such as **Picture Show, Medical Scramble,** and **Medical Detective** (on the CD-ROM) bring new relevance and reinforcement to your study. **Matching Exercises** added to *Appendix I* (Body Systems) will help and test your comprehension of that material.

My major goal is to present an introduction and overview of medical language, with emphasis on basic, essential terminology. Although the text has been updated and carefully reviewed for clarity, simplicity, and practicality, its essential elements remain. Here are its important features:

WORKBOOK-TEXT FORMAT. You learn by interaction and writing terms—completing exercise questions, labeling diagrams, testing your understanding with review sheets, and practicing pronunciation and comprehension of terms. Learning is a complex process. The best path to success is to write terms and their meanings as you test yourself.

EASY TO READ AND UNDERSTAND. I do not assume any background knowledge of biology or medicine. Explanations of terms are worded simply and clearly, and repetition reinforces learning throughout the text. Answers to questions are easily located so that you can check and correct your responses while gaining additional explanation of terminology.

INTRODUCTION TO BODY SYSTEMS. *Appendix I* (Body Systems) includes the following five sections:

1. **Anatomy**—shows full-color images of each body system, labeled for easy reference with combining forms for each body part.

2. **Terminology**—repeats each combining form and gives a medical term illustrating the use of the combining form. Meanings are easily found in the *Glossary of Medical Terms* at the end of the book.

3. **Pathology**—presents explanations of disease conditions related to each body system.

4. **Diagnostic and Treatment Procedures**—explains and defines common examples for each system.

5. **Matching Exercises**—test your understanding of the material, with answers included.

REFERENCE GUIDE FOR MEDICAL AND HOSPITAL WORK. *Appendix II* is a list of **Diagnostic Tests and Procedures** (radiological, nuclear medicine, and clinical and laboratory tests) that you will encounter in the workplace. *Appendix III* contains **Abbreviations, Symbols, and Acronyms** that are in common use. The *Glossary of Medical Terms* is a **mini-dictionary**, designed to help you as you study each chapter. A *Glossary of Word Parts* and *Glossary of English → Spanish Terms* (with images of the body and parts labeled in Spanish) are additional useful references.

PRACTICAL APPLICATIONS. Throughout the text, and especially included in the newly expanded **CD-ROM**, you will find exciting images, practical applications, and medical vignettes that illustrate terminology in the context of stories about patients and procedures. **Medical Detective** is a new feature on the CD-ROM. A medical case is presented, and you answer questions to test your understanding of the situation.

AUDIO GLOSSARY. Pronunciation of terminology for each chapter and an overall audio glossary give you additional practice in hearing and pronouncing terms (on the CD-ROM).

Medical Terminology: A Short Course is exactly what you need to begin your medical career—whether in an office, hospital, or other medical setting. Use this handy book in a classroom with an instructor or study it on your own. The combination of visually reinforced hands-on learning plus easily accessible reference material will mean success for you in your allied health career.

After 30+ years teaching medical terminology, I know this method will work for you. I am available for help at any time. Please communicate your comments, questions, and suggestions to me at MedDavi@aol.com. For technical assistance, please contact technical.support@elsevier.com.

Most of all, I hope this book brings excitement and enthusiasm for the medical language. It can ignite your imagination for new challenges and make your job more interesting. Work hard and have fun learning medical terminology!

Davi-Ellen Chabner

Acknowledgments

Thanks first to my incomparable editor, Maureen Pfeifer, whose intelligent and perceptive advice is evident in every aspect of this edition. I value and rely on her keen insight and willingness to help in all matters related to my work.

Becky Swisher, developmental editor, Health Professions II Editorial, and Christina Pryor, editorial assistant, Health Professions II Editorial, contributed with conscientious, skillful, and reliable hard work. Thanks, Becky, for your unwavering support and responsiveness to any question or task. Anne Altepeter, senior project manager, Book Production, coordinated production of this edition with great care and superb attention to detail.

Ellen Zanolle, senior book designer, Art/Design, created the dynamic cover and interior design, and skillfully executed page layouts. She has been a devoted and enthusiastic partner through other editions as well. Thank you, Ellen!

I am grateful for the confidence, hard work, and cooperation that I have received from Elsevier. In particular, I thank Andrew Allen, publishing director, Health Professions II Editorial; Jeanne Wilke, executive editor, Health Professions II Editorial; Peggy Fagen, director of publishing services, Book Production; Patricia Tannian, publishing services manager, Book Production; Tina Kult, multimedia producer, Multimedia Production; Kim Hamby, product manager, Marketing; and Sharon Salomon, creative director, Creative Services.

Thanks to Jim Perkins, assistant professor of medical illustration, Rochester Institute of Technology, for creating the outstanding images to illustrate terminology throughout this edition.

I appreciated the valuable insights of the instructors who reviewed *Medical Terminology: A Short Course* for this new edition. They are listed with their credentials on a separate page. Their helpful comments are incorporated in the text.

Teachers and students continue to contact me with relevant questions and insights. Thank you to instructors Eileen Streight, Susan Webb, Kathy Trawick, Joanne Williams, Alan Rosenberg, Jim Dresbach, Heather Prutzman, Julie McClure, Denise Tonkinson, Victoria Figueroa, Joyce Nakano, Lynn Scott, and Jackie Benson. Thank you to students Brenda Fox, Alfredo Escobar, Marie Giveleghian, Peggy Mangus, Tom Craig, and Cheryl Revus.

I am grateful to my husband, Bruce Chabner, M.D., and daughter, Elizabeth Chabner Thompson, M.D., M.P.H., who are always available for expert medical advice and editing. Daily visits with my 86-year-old mother, Estelle Rosenzweig, teach me much about the acute and chronic health issues of the elderly. Her strong spirit, resilience, and encouragement are motivating forces reminding me of life's fragility and the importance of making every day count.

Davi-Ellen Chabner

Contents

1

Basic Word Structure

Chapter Sections

Chapter Objectives

- To divide medical terms into component parts
- To analyze, pronounce, and spell medical terms using common combining forms, suffixes, and prefixes

I. **Word Analysis**

If you work in a medical setting, you use medical words every day. As a consumer and citizen, you hear medical terms in your doctor's office, read about health issues in the newspaper, and make daily decisions about your own health care and the health care of your family. Terms such as arthritis, electrocardiogram, hepatitis, and anemia describe conditions and tests that are familiar. Other medical words are more complicated, but as you work in this book, you will begin to understand them even if you have never studied biology or science.

Medical words are like individual jigsaw puzzles. Once you divide the terms into their component parts and learn the meaning of the individual parts, you can use that knowledge to understand many other new terms.

For example, the term HEMATOLOGY is divided into three parts:

When you analyze a medical term, begin at the end of the word. The ending is called a **suffix.** All medical terms contain suffixes. The suffix in HEMATOLOGY is -LOGY, which means study of. Now look at the beginning of the term. HEMAT- is the word **root.** The root gives the essential meaning of the term. The root HEMAT- means blood.

The third part of this term, which is the letter O, has no meaning of its own but is an important connector between the root (HEMAT-) and the suffix (-LOGY). It is called a **combining vowel.** The letter O is the combining vowel usually found in medical terms.

Putting together the meaning of the suffix and the root, the term HEMATOLOGY means the study of blood.

Here is another familiar medical term: ELECTROCARDIOGRAM. You probably know this term, often abbreviated as EKG or ECG. This is how you divide it into its parts:

Start with the **suffix** at the end of the term. The suffix -GRAM means a record.

Now look at the beginning of the term. ELECTR- is a word **root,** and it means electricity.

This medical term has two roots. The second root is CARDI-, meaning heart. Whenever you see CARDI- in other medical terms, you will know that it means heart. ***Read the meaning of medical terms from the suffix, back to the beginning of the term, then across.*** Thus the entire term means record of the electricity in the heart. It is the electricity flowing within the heart that causes the heart muscle to contract, pumping blood throughout your body. The contraction and relaxation of heart muscle are called the heartbeat.

Notice the two combining vowels in ELECTROCARDIOGRAM. Looking for the O in medical terms will help you divide the term into its parts. One combining vowel (O) lies between roots (ELECTR- and CARDI-), and another between the root (CARDI-) and suffix (-GRAM).

The combining vowel *plus* the root is called a **combining form.** For example, there are *two* combining forms in the word ELECTROCARDIOGRAM. These combining forms are ELECTR/O, meaning electricity, and CARDI/O, meaning heart.

Notice how the following medical term is analyzed. Can you locate the two combining forms in this term?

GASTR/O/ENTER/O/LOGY

root	**root**	**suffix**
(stomach)	(intestines)	(study of)

The two combining forms are GASTR/O and ENTER/O. The entire word (reading from the suffix, back to the beginning of the term, and across) means study of the stomach and the intestines. Here are other words that are divided into component parts:

GASTR/O/SCOPE

combining form (stomach) **suffix** (instrument to visually examine)

means instrument to visually examine the stomach.

GASTR/IC

root (stomach) **suffix** (pertaining to)

means pertaining to the stomach. Notice that the combining vowel is dropped when the suffix (-IC) begins with a vowel. Words ending in -IC are adjectives and mean pertaining to.

CARDI/AC

root (heart) **suffix** (pertaining to)

means pertaining to the heart. Again, the combining vowel is dropped when the suffix (-AC) begins with a vowel. Words ending in -AC are adjectives and mean pertaining to.

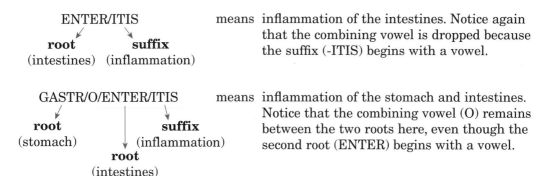

ENTER/ITIS

root (intestines) suffix (inflammation)

means inflammation of the intestines. Notice again that the combining vowel is dropped because the suffix (-ITIS) begins with a vowel.

GASTR/O/ENTER/ITIS

root (stomach) suffix (inflammation) root (intestines)

means inflammation of the stomach and intestines. Notice that the combining vowel (O) remains between the two roots here, even though the second root (ENTER) begins with a vowel.

In addition to roots, suffixes, combining forms, and combining vowels, many medical terms have a word part attached to the *beginning* of the term. This is called a **prefix,** and it can change the meaning of a term in important ways. For example, watch what happens to the meaning of the following medical terms when the prefix changes:

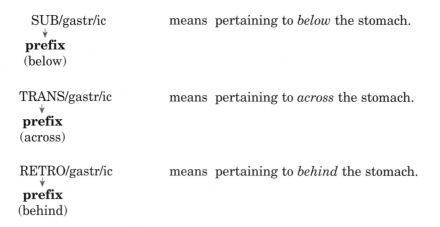

SUB/gastr/ic

prefix (below)

means pertaining to *below* the stomach.

TRANS/gastr/ic

prefix (across)

means pertaining to *across* the stomach.

RETRO/gastr/ic

prefix (behind)

means pertaining to *behind* the stomach.

Let's **review** the important word parts:
1. **Root**—gives the essential *meaning* of the term.
2. **Suffix**—is the word *ending*.
3. **Prefix**—is a small part added to the *beginning* of a term.
4. **Combining vowel**—*connects* roots to suffixes and roots to other roots.
5. **Combining form**—is the combination of the *root* and the *combining vowel*.

Some important rules to **remember** are:
1. **Read** the meaning of medical words from the suffix to the beginning of the word and then across.
2. **Drop** the combining vowel before a suffix that starts with a vowel.
3. **Keep** the combining vowel between word roots, even if the root begins with a vowel.

II. Combining Forms, Suffixes, and Prefixes

Here is a list of combining forms, suffixes, and prefixes that are commonly found in medical terms. Write the meaning of the medical term on the line that is provided. There will be terms that are more difficult to understand even after you write the meanings of individual word parts. For these, more extensive explanations are given in italics. To check your work, see the *Glossary of Medical Terms,* which contains meanings of all terms and can be found on p. 313.

In your study of medical terminology, you will find it helpful to practice writing terms and their meanings many times. Complete the Exercises in Section III, the Review in Section IV, and the Pronunciation of Terms list in Section V as you begin your study of the medical language.

Combining Forms

Notice that the combining form is bolded, and the root in the medical term is underlined.

Combining Form	Meaning	Medical Term	Meaning
aden/o	gland	<u>aden</u>oma _____ -OMA *means tumor or mass.*	
		<u>aden</u>itis _____ -ITIS *means inflammation.*	
arthr/o	joint	<u>arthr</u>itis _____	
bi/o	life	<u>bi</u>ology _____ -LOGY *means study of.*	
		<u>bi</u>opsy _____ -OPSY *means to view. Living tissue is removed and viewed under a microscope.*	
carcin/o	cancer, cancerous	<u>carcin</u>oma _____	
cardi/o	heart	<u>cardi</u>ology _____	
cephal/o	head	<u>cephal</u>ic _____ -IC *means pertaining to.*	

cerebr/o   cerebrum, largest part of the brain

cerebral _____

-AL means pertaining to. Figure 1-1 shows the cerebrum and its functions.

cerebrovascular accident (CVA) _____

-VASCULAR means pertaining to blood vessels; a CVA is commonly known as a stroke.

cyst/o   urinary bladder

cystoscope _____

-SCOPE means instrument to visually examine. Figure 1-2 shows the urinary bladder and urinary tract. A cystoscope is placed through the urethra into the urinary bladder. See Figure 1-3.

Sensations from body — Movement — Writing — Hearing — Vision — Reading — Spinal cord — Eye movement — Thought processes — Smell — Speech

FIGURE 1–1

The cerebrum and its functions.

FIGURE 1–2

The urinary tract. (Modified from Chabner D-E: *The Language of Medicine,* ed 7, Philadelphia, 2004, WB Saunders.)

FIGURE 1–3

A **cystoscope** is placed into the urinary bladder through the urethra within the penis. (Modified from Chabner D-E: *The Language of Medicine,* ed 7, Philadelphia, 2004, WB Saunders.)

1

cyt/o	cell	cytology _____

**dermat/o,
derm/o**   skin   dermatitis _____

dermal _____

electr/o   electricity   electrocardiogram (ECG, EKG) _____
-GRAM *means record.*

encephal/o   brain   electroencephalogram (EEG) _____
*This record is helpful in determining whether a patient
has a seizure disorder, such as epilepsy.*

enter/o   intestines
(often the
small
intestine)   enteritis _____
*Figure 1-4 shows the small and large intestines.
ENTER/O describes the small intestine and sometimes
intestines in general. COL/O and COLON/O are combining
forms for the large intestine (colon).*

erythr/o   red   erythrocyte _____
*-CYTE means cell. Figure 1-5 shows the three major types
of blood cells.*

gastr/o   stomach   gastroscopy _____
*-SCOPY means process of visual examination using an
instrument, or "scope."*

gnos/o   knowledge   diagnosis _____
*-SIS means state of; DIA- means complete. A diagnosis is
the complete knowledge gained after testing and examining
the patient. The plural of diagnosis is diagnoses. Table 1-1
on p. 11 shows other plural formations.*

prognosis _____
*PRO- means before. A prognosis is a prediction (before
knowledge) that is actually made after the diagnosis. It
forecasts the outcome of treatment.*

gynec/o   woman,
female   gynecology _____

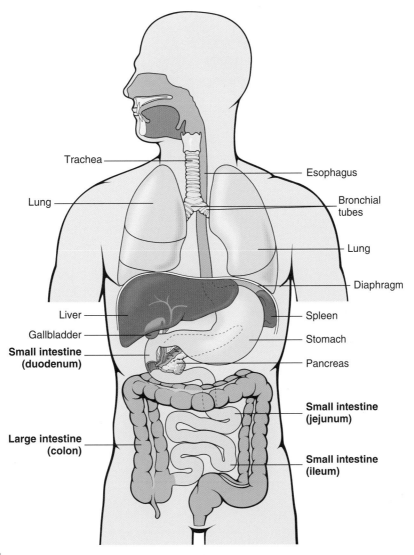

FIGURE 1–4

Location of the small and large intestines in the abdominal cavity. Note that the lungs, bronchial tubes, trachea, and esophagus are in the chest cavity, which is above the diaphragm. (Modified from Chabner D-E: *The Language of Medicine,* ed 7, Philadelphia, 2004, WB Saunders.)

ERYTHROCYTES

(side view)

LEUKOCYTES

1. Eosinophil   2. Basophil   3. Neutrophil

4. Lymphocyte   5. Monocyte

THROMBOCYTES (PLATELETS)

FIGURE 1–5

Blood cells: *erythrocytes* (carry oxygen), ***leukocytes*** (five different types help fight disease), and ***thrombocytes*** or ***platelets*** (help blood to clot). (Modified from Chabner D-E: *The Language of Medicine,* ed 7, Philadelphia, 2004, WB Saunders.)

hemat/o, hem/o	blood	hematoma _____
		-OMA *means mass or tumor. In this term, -oma indicates a mass or swelling containing blood. A hematoma is a bruise or "black-and-blue" mark.*
		hemoglobin _____
		-GLOBIN *means protein. Hemoglobin is the protein in red blood cells (erythrocytes) that helps carry oxygen in the blood.*
hepat/o	liver	hepatitis _____

TABLE 1–1	FORMATION OF PLURALS

Consult the *Glossary of Medical Terms* for pronunciations of all terms.

1. Words ending in **a,** retain the **a** and add **e:**

SINGULAR	PLURAL	MEANING
vertebra	vertebrae	Backbones
bursa	bursae	Sacs of fluid near a joint

2. Words ending in **is,** drop the **is** and add **es:**

SINGULAR	PLURAL	MEANING
diagnosis	diagnoses	Determinations of the nature and cause of diseases
psychosis	psychoses	Abnormal conditions of the mind

3. Words ending in **ex** or **ix,** drop the **ex** or **ix,** and add **ices:**

SINGULAR	PLURAL	MEANING
apex	apices	Pointed ends of organs
cortex	cortices	Outer parts of organs
varix	varices	Enlarged, swollen veins

4. Words ending in **on,** drop the **on** and add **a:**

SINGULAR	PLURAL	MEANING
ganglion	ganglia	Groups of nerve cells; benign cysts near a joint (such as the wrist)

5. Words ending in **um,** drop the **um** and add **a:**

SINGULAR	PLURAL	MEANING
bacterium	bacteria	Types of one-celled organisms
ovum	ova	Egg cells

6. Words ending in **us,** drop the **us** and add **i*:**

SINGULAR	PLURAL	MEANING
bronchus	bronchi	Tubes leading from the windpipe to the lungs
calculus	calculi	Stones

*Exceptions to this rule are viruses and sinuses.

lapar/o	abdomen (area between the chest and hip)	laparotomy _____ -TOMY *means incision (to cut into). An exploratory laparotomy is a large incision of the abdominal wall made to inspect abdominal organs for evidence of disease. Another combining form for abdomen is* ABDOMIN/O, *as in abdominal.*
leuk/o	white	leukocyte _____ *Figure 1-5 shows five different types of leukocytes.*
nephr/o	kidney	nephrectomy _____ -ECTOMY *means to cut out; an excision or resection of an organ or part of the body.*
neur/o	nerve	neurology _____

1

onc/o	tumor	oncologist _____	

-IST means a specialist.

ophthalm/o   eye   ophthalmoscope _____

Figure 1-6 shows an ophthalmologist examining a patient with an ophthalmoscope.

oste/o   bone   osteoarthritis _____

Figure 1-7 shows a normal knee joint and a knee joint with osteoarthritis. Degenerative changes and loss of cartilage occur. Inflammation of the joint membrane occurs late in the disease.

path/o   disease   pathologist _____

A pathologist is a medical doctor who views biopsy samples to make a diagnosis and examines a dead body (in an autopsy) to determine the cause of death. AUT- means self, and -OPSY means to view. Thus an autopsy is an opportunity to see for oneself what has happened to the patient to cause his or her death.

psych/o   mind   psychosis _____

-OSIS means abnormal condition. This is a serious mental condition in which the patient loses touch with reality.

Viewing aperture

Disk for changing lenses

Light

FIGURE 1–6

Ophthalmoscope. It allows the ophthalmologist to view the outer and inner areas of the eye. (Modified from Chabner D-E: *The Language of Medicine,* ed 7, Philadelphia, 2004, WB Saunders.)

FIGURE 1–7

Normal knee joint and knee joint with **osteoarthritis.**

| **ren/o** | kidney | renal _____ |

Sometimes there are two combining forms for the same part of the body. One comes from Latin, and the other from Greek (REN- is the Latin root meaning "kidney," and NEPHR- is the Greek root meaning "kidney"). The Greek root describes abnormal conditions and procedures, whereas the Latin root is used with -AL, meaning "pertaining to."

| **rhin/o** | nose | rhinitis _____ |

| **sarc/o** | flesh | sarcoma _____ |

Sarcomas and carcinomas are cancerous tumors. Sarcomas grow from the fleshy tissues of the body, such as muscle, fat, bone, and cartilage, whereas carcinomas arise from skin tissue and the linings of internal organs.

| **thromb/o** | clotting | thrombocyte _____ |

*A thrombocyte **(platelet)** is a small cell that helps blood to clot. Platelets are shown in Figure 1-5.*

thrombosis _____

*A **thrombus** (blood clot) occurs when thrombocytes and other clotting factors combine. **Thrombosis** describes the condition of forming a clot (thrombus).*

Suffixes

Suffix	Meaning	Medical Term	Meaning
-al	pertaining to	neur<u>al</u> _____	
		Other suffixes meaning pertaining to are found in Chapter 3, p. 85.	
-algia	pain	arthr<u>algia</u> _____	
-cyte	cell	leuko<u>cyte</u> _____	
-ectomy	cutting out; removal, excision	gastr<u>ectomy</u> _____	
		In a partial or subtotal gastrectomy, only a portion of the stomach is removed.	
-emia	blood condition	leuk<u>emia</u> _____	
		Large numbers of immature, cancerous cells are found in the bloodstream and bone marrow (inner part of bone that makes blood cells).	
-globin	protein	hemo<u>globin</u> _____	
-gram	record	arthro<u>gram</u> _____	
		This is an x-ray record of a joint.	
-ia	condition	cephal<u>gia</u> _____	
		Notice this term is shortened from cephalalgia.	
-ic	pertaining to	gastr<u>ic</u> _____	
-ism	condition, process	hyperthyroid<u>ism</u> _____	
		HYPER- means excessive. The thyroid gland is in the neck. It secretes the hormone thyroxine, which helps cells burn food to release energy. See Figure 1-8.	
-itis	inflammation	gastroenter<u>itis</u> _____	
-logist	specialist in the	neuro<u>logist</u> _____	
-logy	study of	nephro<u>logy</u> _____	
		See Table 1-2 for a list of other terms using -LOGY.	

FIGURE 1–8

Hyperthyroidism. The thyroid gland produces too much hormone and causes symptoms such as rapid pulse, nervousness, excessive sweating, and swelling of tissue behind the eyeball (exophthalmos). (Modified from Seidel H et al: *Mosby's Guide to Physical Examination,* ed 4, St Louis, 1998, Mosby.)

-oma	tumor, mass	hepat<u>oma</u> _____
		This is a cancerous (malignant) tumor also called ***hepatocellular carcinoma.***
-opsy	to view	bi<u>opsy</u> _____
-osis	abnormal condition	nephr<u>osis</u> _____

TABLE 1–2	TERMS USING -LOGY (STUDY OF)
cardiology	Study of the heart
dermatology	Study of the skin
endocrinology	Study of the endocrine glands
gastroenterology	Study of the stomach and intestines
gynecology	Study of women and women's disease
hematology	Study of the blood
neurology	Study of the nerves and the brain and spinal cord
oncology	Study of tumors (cancerous or malignant diseases)
ophthalmology	Study of the eye
pathology	Study of disease
psychology	Study of the mind and mental disorders
rheumatology	Study of joint diseases (RHEUMAT/O means flow or watery discharge, which was once thought to cause aches and pains, especially in joints.)

-scope   instrument to   gastro<u>scope</u> _____
                  visually examine

-scopy   process of visual   lapar<u>oscopy</u> _____
                  examination

Small incisions are made near the navel, and instruments are inserted into the abdomen for viewing organs and performing procedures such as tying off the fallopian tubes. See Figure 1-9.

                                            arthr<u>oscopy</u> _____

See Figure 1-10.

-sis   state of   progno<u>sis</u> _____

-tomy   process of cutting   neuro<u>tomy</u> _____
                  into; incision

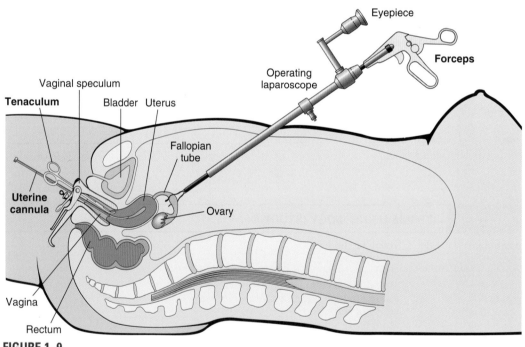

FIGURE 1–9

Laparoscopy for tubal ligation (interruption of the continuity of the fallopian tubes) as a means of preventing future pregnancy. The **_tenaculum_** keeps the vaginal cavity open. The **_uterine cannula_** is a tube placed into the uterus to move the uterus during the procedure. **_Forceps,_** placed through the laparoscope, are used for grasping or manipulating tissue. (Modified from Chabner D-E: *The Language of Medicine,* ed 7, Philadelphia, 2004, WB Saunders.)

FIGURE 1–10

Arthroscopy of the knee.

Prefixes

Prefixes	Meaning	Medical Term	Meaning
a-, an-	no, not	anemia _____	
		Literally, anemia means a condition of "no blood." Actually, it is a decrease in the number of red blood cells or a decrease in their ability to carry oxygen because of less hemoglobin, a protein that helps carry oxygen in red blood cells.	
aut-	self	autopsy _____	
		Viewing and examining a dead body with one's own (self) eyes.	
dia-	complete, through	diagnosis _____	
dys-	bad, painful, difficult, abnormal	dysentery _____	
		The suffix -Y means condition or process.	

1

endo-	within	endocrine glands _____

*CRIN/O means to secrete (to form and give off). Examples of endocrine glands are the thyroid gland, pituitary gland, adrenal glands, ovaries, and testes. All these glands secrete hormones **within** the body and into the bloodstream.*

endocardium _____

The valves and chambers within the heart are lined with endocardium.

exo-	outside	exocrine glands _____

*Examples of exocrine glands are sweat, tear, and mammary (breast) glands that secrete substances to the **outside** of the body.*

hyper-	excessive, more than normal, too much	hyperglycemia _____

GLYC/O- means sugar. Hyperglycemia is also known as diabetes mellitus. Mellitus means "sweet."

hypo-	below, less than normal, under	hypodermic _____

A hypodermic syringe (an instrument for injecting or withdrawing fluid) is placed under the skin. See Figure 1-11.

hypoglycemia _____

FIGURE 1–11

A **hypodermic syringe** inserted under the skin.

pro-	before	prognosis _____

re-	back	resection _____

-SECTION means to cut into an organ, but RESECTION *means to cut an organ out in the sense of cutting back or away. The Latin* resectio *means "a trimming or pruning."*

retro-	behind	retrogastric _____

sub-	below, under	subhepatic _____

trans-	across, through	transdermal _____

transurethral _____

The urethra is a tube that leads from the urinary bladder to the outside of the body. See Figure 1-2.

III. Exercises and Answers

These exercises give you practice writing and understanding the terms presented in Section II. An important part of your work is to *check your answers* with the answer key beginning on p. 27. If you cannot answer a question, then please look at the answer key and *copy* the correct answer. You may want to photocopy some of the exercises before you complete them so that you can practice doing them many times.

A. Using slashes (/), divide the following terms into their component parts and give the meaning for the whole term. The first term is completed as an example:

1. aden/oma   *Tumor of a gland* _____

2. arthritis _____

3. biopsy _____

4. cardiology _____

5. dermal _____

6. cytology _____

7. cystoscope _____

8. cerebral _____

9. cephalic _____

10. adenitis _____

B. Complete the following sentences using the medical terms given below:

diagnosis	erythrocyte	hepatitis
electrocardiogram	gynecology	prognosis
electroencephalogram	hematoma	
enteritis	hemoglobin	

1. A mass of blood, or "black-and-blue" mark, is a(an) _____.

2. A red blood cell is a(an) _____.

3. Inflammation of the small intestine is _____.

4. The prediction about the outcome of an illness is a(an) _____.

5. The record of electricity in the brain is a(an) _____.

6. The process of study of women and women's disease is _____.

7. The record of electricity in the heart is a(an) _____.

8. Complete knowledge of a patient's illness on the basis of tests and other

   information is a(an) _____.

9. A protein found in red blood cells is _____.

10. Inflammation of the liver is _____.

C. Name the part of the body described in the following terms and give the meaning of the entire term:

1. laparotomy _____

2. nephrectomy _____

3. neuritis _____

4. ophthalmoscope _____

5. osteotomy _____

6. renal _____

7. rhinitis _____

8. sarcoma _____

D. Give the meanings of the following terms:

1. oncologist _____

2. pathologist _____

3. psychosis _____

4. leukocyte _____

5. thrombocyte _____

6. gastritis _____

7. adenoma _____

8. thrombosis _____

E. Give the meaning of the following suffixes:

1. -cyte _____

2. -ism _____

3. -ectomy _____

4. -al _____

5. -emia _____

6. -gram _____

7. -algia _____

8. -itis _____

9. -globin _____

10. -ic _____

1

F. Complete the following medical terms to end each sentence.

1. Removal of a nerve is **neur** _____.

2. Large numbers of immature, cancerous white blood cells is a blood condition known

   as **leuk** _____.

3. An x-ray record of a joint is **arthro** _____.

4. Study of the kidney is **nephro** _____.

5. Tumor of the liver is **hepat** _____.

6. Visual examination of the abdomen is **laparo** _____.

7. An incision of a joint is called **arthro** _____.

8. Abnormal condition of the skin is **dermat** _____.

9. Inflammation of the skin is **dermat** _____.

10. A specialist in the study of blood is a **hemato** _____.

G. Give the meanings of the following prefixes:

1. hyper- _____

2. sub- _____

3. dys- _____

4. trans- _____

5. retro- _____

6. dia- _____

7. exo- _____

8. aut- _____

9. hypo- _____

10. endo- _____

H. Give meanings of the following medical terms:

1. autopsy _____

2. hyperthyroidism _____

3. anemia _____

4. dysentery _____

5. endocrine glands _____

6. hypoglycemia _____

7. exocrine glands _____

8. resection _____

9. transdermal _____

10. hyperglycemia _____

I. Complete the following medical terms related to the stomach:

1. _____gastric   Pertaining to **under** the stomach.

2. gastr_____   **Pain** in the stomach.

3. gastr_____   **Inflammation** of the stomach.

4. _____gastric   Pertaining to **across** or **through** the stomach.

5. gastr_____   **Process of visually examining** the stomach.

6. _____gastric   Pertaining to **behind** the stomach.

   7. gastr_____   **Study of** the stomach and intestines.

   8. gastr_____   **Incision** of the stomach.

   9. gastr_____   **Excision** of the stomach.

   10. gastr_____   **Instrument to visually examine** the stomach.

J. On the line provided, give the meaning of the bolded term:

   1. An **oncologist** treats abnormal conditions such as sarcomas and carcinomas.

   _____

   2. After explaining the diagnosis, Dr. Jones outlined the treatment and assured the

   patient that the **prognosis** was hopeful. _____

   _____

   3. Elderly Mrs. Scott has constant arthralgias in her knees and hips. Her physician

   prescribes anti-inflammatory drugs and aspirin to treat her **osteoarthritis** but

   advises that joint replacement may be necessary. _____

   _____

   4. A **pathologist** is a medical doctor who performs autopsies and examines biopsy

   samples. _____

   5. **Thrombosis** is a serious condition that may result in blockage of blood vessels.

   _____

   6. **Hyperglycemia** results from lack of insulin (hormone) secretion from the pancreas

   (an endocrine gland near the stomach). Without insulin, sugar cannot enter cells

   and remains in the blood. _____

   _____

7. Schizophrenia is an example of a **psychosis** in which the patient loses touch with reality and displays abnormal behavior. _____

_____

8. Minimally invasive surgery of the abdomen is known as **laparoscopy.** With this procedure, the gallbladder and appendix may be removed with instruments inserted into small incisions. _____

_____

9. Symptoms of **hyperthyroidism** include an enlarged thyroid gland and protruding eyeballs (exophthalmos). _____

_____

10. Sally's diagnosis of **dysentery** was made after she returned from a trip to Mexico with abdominal pain, fever, and severe diarrhea (loose, watery stools).

_____

11. Mr. Smith died of a **cerebrovascular accident.** Confirmation at autopsy revealed a thrombus blocking one of his cerebral arteries. _____

_____

12. **Erythrocytes** contain hemoglobin that enables them to carry oxygen throughout the body. _____

13. **Leukemia** was confirmed after a bone marrow biopsy and high white blood cell counts. _____

14. Certain types of bleeding or clotting disorders may be caused by reduced numbers of thrombocytes, also known as **platelets.** _____

15. An example of **anemia** is iron-deficiency anemia. _____

_____

16. **Transdermal** delivery by patch is used for administering drugs such as nicotine,

nitroglycerin, and scopolamine (for motion sickness). _____

_____

K. Refer to Table 1-1 to form the plurals of the following terms:

1. psychosis _____

2. ovum _____

3. vertebra _____

4. bronchus _____

5. spermatozoon _____

6. apex _____

L. Circle the term that best completes the meaning of the sentences in the following medical vignettes:

1. Selma ate a spicy meal at an Indian restaurant. Later that night she experienced **(osteoarthritis, dermatitis, gastroenteritis).** Fortunately the cramping and diarrhea subsided by morning.

2. Christina was feeling very sluggish, both physically and mentally. Her hair seemed coarse, she had noticed weight gain in the past weeks, and she had hot and cold intolerance, never really feeling comfortable. Her internist referred her to a gland specialist, a(an) **(gynecologist, endocrinologist, pathologist).** The physician ordered a blood test that revealed low levels of a hormone from a gland in her neck. The diagnosis of **(hypothyroidism, hyperthyroidism, psychosis)** was thus made, and proper treatment prescribed.

3. Dr. Fischer examined the lump in Bruno's thigh. An imaging technique using magnetic waves and radio signals (MRI scan) revealed a suspicious mass in the soft connective tissue of the thigh. Suspecting a cancerous mass of flesh tissue, or **(hematoma, carcinoma, sarcoma),** Dr. Fischer suggested a(an) **(prognosis, biopsy, autopsy)** of the mass.

4. On her seventh birthday, Susie fell down during her birthday party. Her mother noticed bruises on Susie's knees and elbows that seemed to come up "over night." Her pediatrician ordered a blood test that demonstrated decreased platelet count and elevated **(leukocyte, erythrocyte, thrombocyte)** count at 40,000 cells. Susie was referred to a(an) **(dermatologist, nephrologist, oncologist)** who made a diagnosis of **(hepatitis, anemia, leukemia).**

5. When Mr. Saluto collapsed and died while eating dinner, the family requested a(an) **(laparotomy, gastroscopy, autopsy)** to determine the cause of death. The **(hematologist, pathologist, gastroenterologist)** discovered that Mr. Saluto had died of a **(cardiovascular accident, dysentery, cerebrovascular accident),** otherwise known as a stroke.

Answers to Exercises

A

1. Tumor of a gland
2. Inflammation of a joint
3. Process of viewing living tissue under a microscope
4. Study of (process of study of) the heart
5. Pertaining to the skin
6. Study of (process of study of) cells
7. Instrument to visually examine the urinary bladder
8. Pertaining to the cerebrum (largest part of the brain)
9. Pertaining to the head
10. Inflammation of a gland

B

1. hematoma
2. erythrocyte
3. enteritis
4. prognosis
5. electroencephalogram
6. gynecology
7. electrocardiogram
8. diagnosis
9. hemoglobin
10. hepatitis

C

1. abdomen: incision of the abdomen (this is also called exploratory surgery).
2. kidney: excision (removal, resection) of the kidney.
3. nerve: inflammation of a nerve.
4. eye: instrument to visually examine the eye.
5. bone: incision (cut into, section) of a bone.
6. kidney: pertaining to the kidney.
7. nose: inflammation of the nose.
8. flesh tissue: tumor (cancerous or malignant) of flesh tissue.

D

1. Specialist in the study of tumors (cancerous or malignant tumors)
2. Specialist in the study of disease (examines biopsy samples and performs autopsies)
3. Abnormal condition of the mind
4. White blood cell
5. Clotting cell or platelet
6. Inflammation of the stomach
7. Tumor of a gland (this is a benign or harmless tumor). An adenocarcinoma is a malignant tumor (CARCIN/O means cancerous)
8. Abnormal condition of clotting (occurring in a blood vessel)

E

1. cell
2. condition, process
3. process of cutting out, excision, resection, removal
4. pertaining to
5. condition of blood (blood condition)
6. record
7. pain; condition of pain
8. inflammation
9. protein
10. pertaining to

F

1. neurectomy
2. leukemia
3. arthrogram
4. nephrology
5. hepatoma or hepatocellular carcinoma
6. laparoscopy
7. arthrotomy
8. dermatosis
9. dermatitis
10. hematologist

G

1. excessive, above, more than normal
2. under, below
3. abnormal, bad, difficult, painful
4. across, through
5. behind, back
6. complete, through
7. out, outside
8. self
9. below, deficient, less than normal
10. within, in, inner

H

1. Examination of a dead body to determine the cause of death
2. Excessive activity of the thyroid gland
3. Deficiency of hemoglobin or numbers of red blood cells; literally "no" (AN-) "blood" (-EMIA)
4. Condition of painful intestine; marked by inflammation, abdominal pain, frequent and bloody stools and often caused by bacteria
5. Organs that produce (secrete) hormones directly into the bloodstream
6. Blood condition of decreased sugar (lower than normal levels)
7. Organs that produce (secrete) chemicals to the outside of the body (through tubes or ducts)
8. Removal (excision) of an organ or structure
9. Pertaining to through the skin
10. Blood condition of increased sugar (higher than normal levels)

I

1. subgastric or hypogastric
2. gastralgia
3. gastritis
4. transgastric
5. gastroscopy
6. retrogastric
7. gastroenterology
8. gastrotomy
9. gastrectomy
10. gastroscope

J

1. Specialist in the study (and treatment) of tumors
2. Prediction of the outcome of an illness or treatment
3. Inflammation of bones and joints (including degeneration of joints)
4. Specialist in the study of disease
5. Abnormal condition of clotting (clot formation)
6. Blood condition of increased sugar
7. Abnormal condition of the mind
8. Visual examination of the abdomen
9. Condition of increased secretion of hormone from the thyroid gland
10. Condition of painful intestines
11. Disorder of blood vessels within the cerebrum; stroke
12. Red blood cells
13. Increase in cancerous (malignant) white blood cells in blood and bone marrow
14. Clotting cells
15. Deficiency of hemoglobin and/or numbers of red blood cells; resulting in reduced oxygen to cells
16. Pertaining to through the skin

K

1. psychos**es** (drop **-is** and add **-es**)
2. ov**a** (drop **-um** and add **-a**)
3. vertebra**e** (add **-e**)
4. bronch**i** (drop **-us** and add **-i**)
5. spermatozo**a** (drop **-on** and add **-a**)
6. ap**ices** (drop **-ex** and add **-ices**)

L

1. gastroenteritis
2. endocrinologist, hypothyroidism
3. sarcoma, biopsy
4. leukocyte, oncologist, leukemia
5. autopsy, pathologist, cerebrovascular accident

1

IV. Review

Here is your chance to test your understanding of all the **combining forms, suffixes,** and **prefixes** that you have studied in this chapter. Write the meaning of each term in the space provided and *check* your answers with the answer key at the end of the section on p. 32. All the meanings for word parts are found in the *Glossary of Word Parts* beginning on p. 347.

Combining Forms

Combining Form	Meaning	Combining Form	Meaning
1. aden/o		18. gnos/o	
2. arthr/o		19. gynec/o	
3. bi/o		20. hemat/o, hem/o	
4. carcin/o		21. hepat/o	
5. cardi/o		22. lapar/o	
6. cephal/o		23. leuk/o	
7. cerebr/o		24. nephr/o	
8. crin/o		25. neur/o	
9. cyst/o		26. onc/o	
10. cyt/o		27. ophthalm/o	
11. dermat/o, derm/o		28. oste/o	
12. electr/o		29. path/o	
13. encephal/o		30. psych/o	
14. enter/o		31. rhin/o	
15. erythr/o		32. sarc/o	
16. gastr/o		33. thromb/o	
17. glyc/o			

Suffixes

Suffix	Meaning	Suffix	Meaning
1. -al	_____	11. -logist	_____
2. -algia	_____	12. -logy	_____
3. -cyte	_____	13. -oma	_____
4. -ectomy	_____	14. -opsy	_____
5. -emia	_____	15. -osis	_____
6. -globin	_____	16. -scope	_____
7. -ia	_____	17. -scopy	_____
8. -ic	_____	18. -sis	_____
9. -ism	_____	19. -tomy	_____
10. -itis	_____		

Prefixes

Prefix	Meaning	Prefix	Meaning
1. a-, an-	_____	8. hypo-	_____
2. aut-	_____	9. pro-	_____
3. dia-	_____	10. re-	_____
4. dys-	_____	11. retro-	_____
5. endo-	_____	12. sub-	_____
6. exo-	_____	13. trans-	_____
7. hyper-	_____		

Answers to Review

Combining Forms

1. gland	13. brain	24. kidney
2. joint	14. intestines (often small	25. nerve
3. life	intestine)	26. tumor
4. cancer, cancerous	15. red	27. eye
5. heart	16. stomach	28. bone
6. head	17. sugar	29. disease
7. cerebrum	18. knowledge	30. mind
8. secrete	19. woman, female	31. nose
9. urinary bladder	20. blood	32. flesh
10. cell	21. liver	33. clotting
11. skin	22. abdomen	
12. electricity	23. white	

Suffixes

1. pertaining to	10. inflammation
2. pain	11. specialist in the study of
3. cell	12. study of
4. process of cutting out; removal;	13. tumor, mass
excision	14. to view (process of viewing)
5. blood condition	15. abnormal condition
6. protein	16. instrument to visually examine
7. condition	17. process of visual examination
8. pertaining to	18. state of
9. condition; process	19. process of cutting into; incision

Prefixes

1. no, not	8. below, too little, deficient
2. self	9. before
3. complete	10. back
4. bad, painful, difficult, abnormal	11. behind
5. within	12. under, below
6. out, outside	13. across, through
7. too much, above	

V. Pronunciation of Terms

The terms that you have learned in this chapter are presented here with their pronunciations. The capitalized letters in boldface are the accented syllable. Pronounce each word out loud, then write the meaning in the space provided. All meanings of terms are found in the *Glossary of Medical Terms,* p. 313.

Term	Pronunciation	Meaning
adenitis	ad-eh-**NI**-tis	
adenoma	ah-deh-**NO**-mah	
anemia	ah-**NE**-me-ah	
arthralgia	ar-**THRAL**-jah	
arthritis	ar-**THRI**-tis	
arthrogram	**AR**-thro-gram	
arthroscope	**AR**-thro-skop	
arthroscopy	ar-**THROS**-ko-pe	
autopsy	**AW**-top-se	
biology	bi-**OL**-o-je	
biopsy	**BI**-op-se	
carcinoma	kar-sih-**NO**-mah	
cardiac	**KAR**-de-ak	
cardiology	kar-de-**OL**-o-je	
cephalgia	seh-**FAL**-jah	
cephalic	seh-**FAL**-ik	
cerebral	seh-**RE**-bral	
cerebrovascular accident	seh-re-bro-**VAS**-ku-lar **AK**-sih-dent	

1

cystoscope	**SIS**-to-skop	_____
cystoscopy	sis-**TOS**-ko-pe	_____
cytology	si-**TOL**-o-je	_____
dermal	**DER**-mal	_____
dermatitis	der-mah-**TI**-tis	_____
dermatosis	der-mah-**TO**-sis	_____
diagnosis	di-ag-**NO**-sis	_____
dysentery	**DIS**-en-teh-re	_____
electrocardiogram	e-lek-tro-**KAR**-de-o-gram	_____
electroencephalogram	e-lek-tro-en-**SEF**-ah-lo-gram	_____
endocardium	en-do-**KAR**-de-um	_____
endocrine glands	**EN**-do-krin glanz	_____
endocrinology	en-do-krih-**NOL**-o-je	_____
enteritis	en-teh-**RI**-tis	_____
erythrocyte	eh-**RITH**-ro-site	_____
exocrine glands	**EK**-so-krin glanz	_____
gastrectomy	gas-**TREK**-to-me	_____
gastric	**GAS**-trik	_____
gastritis	gas-**TRI**-tis	_____
gastroenteritis	gas-tro-en-teh-**RI**-tis	_____
gastroenterology	gas-tro-en-ter-**OL**-o-je	_____
gastroscope	**GAS**-tro-skop	_____

gastroscopy	gas-**TROS**-ko-pe _____
gastrotomy	gas-**TROT**-o-me _____
gynecologist	gi-neh-**KOL**-o-jist _____
gynecology	gi-neh-**KOL**-o-je _____
hematoma	he-mah-**TO**-mah _____
hemoglobin	**HE**-mo-glo-bin _____
hepatitis	hep-ah-**TI**-tis _____
hepatoma	hep-ah-**TO**-mah _____
hyperglycemia	hi-per-gli-**SE**-me-ah _____
hyperthyroidism	hi-per-**THI**-royd-izm _____
hypodermic	hi-po-**DER**-mik _____
hypoglycemia	hi-po-gli-**SE**-me-ah _____
hypothyroidism	hi-po-**THI**-royd-izm _____
laparoscopy	lap-ah-**ROS**-ko-pe _____
laparotomy	lap-ah-**ROT**-o-me _____
leukemia	lu-**KE**-me-ah _____
leukocyte	**LU**-ko-site _____
nephrectomy	neh-**FREK**-to-me _____
nephrology	neh-**FROL**-o-je _____
nephrosis	neh-**FRO**-sis _____
neural	**NU**-ral _____
neuralgia	nu-**RAL**-jah _____
neuritis	nu-**RI**-tis _____

1

neurology	nur-**ROL**-o-je _____
neurotomy	nur-**ROT**-o-me _____
oncologist	ong-**KOL**-o-jist _____
ophthalmoscope	of-**THAL**-mo-skop _____
osteitis	os-te-**I**-tis _____
osteoarthritis	os-te-o-ar-**THRI**-tis _____
pathologist	pah-**THOL**-o-jist _____
platelet	**PLAT**-let _____
prognosis	prog-**NO**-sis _____
psychosis	si-**KO**-**sis** _____
renal	**RE**-nal _____
resection	re-**SEK**-shun _____
retrogastric	reh-tro-**GAS**-trik _____
rhinitis	ri-**NI**-tis _____
rhinotomy	ri-**NOT**-o-me _____
sarcoma	sar-**KO**-mah _____
subgastric	sub-**GAS**-trik _____
subhepatic	sub-heh-**PAT**-ik _____
thrombocyte	**THROM**-bo-site _____
thrombosis	throm-**BO**-sis _____
transdermal	trans-**DER**-mal _____
transgastric	trans-**GAS**-trik _____
transurethral	trans-u-**RE**-thral _____

1

VI. Practical Applications

Match the CONDITIONS listed below with PROCEDURES that diagnose or treat each. Write each condition next to its procedure. Answers follow.

Conditions

adenocarcinoma of an endocrine gland in the neck

epilepsy (seizure disorder)

heart attack

leukemia

osteogenic sarcoma (bone cancer)

renal cell carcinoma

stomach ulcer (hollowed out space)

urinary bladder carcinoma

Procedures

1. Below-knee leg resection (amputation) _____

2. Bone marrow biopsy _____

3. Electrocardiogram _____

4. Cystoscopy _____

5. Nephrectomy _____

6. Thyroid gland resection _____

7. Gastroscopy _____

8. Electroencephalogram _____

Answers to Practical Applications

1. osteogenic sarcoma (bone cancer)
2. leukemia
3. heart attack
4. urinary bladder carcinoma
5. renal cell carcinoma

6. adenocarcinoma of an endocrine gland
   in the neck
7. stomach ulcer
8. epilepsy (seizure disorder)

VII. Picture Show

Answer the questions that follow each image. Correct answers are found on p. 40.

A

Blood smear. (Modified from Carr JH, Rodak BF: *Clinical Hematology Atlas,* Philadelphia, 1999, WB Saunders.)

1. The arrows in this photo of a blood smear are pointing to cells that are necessary in blood clotting. These cells are:

   a. leukocytes
   b. thrombosis
   c. platelets
   d. erythrocytes

2. The other blood cells in the photo contain a protein that helps the cell carry oxygen. These cells are:

   a. leukocytes
   b. thrombosis
   c. platelets
   d. erythrocytes

3. The protein contained in the cells is:

   a. hemoglobin
   b. anemia
   c. sarcoma
   d. carcinoma

(Modified from Lewis SM, Heitkemper MM, Dirksen SR: *Medical-Surgical Nursing: Assessment and Management of Clinical Problems,* ed 5, St. Louis, 2004, Mosby.)

1. The image shows a minimally invasive procedure to visually examine the knee. It is:

a. cystoscopy
b. arthroscopy
c. laparoscopy
d. arthrectomy

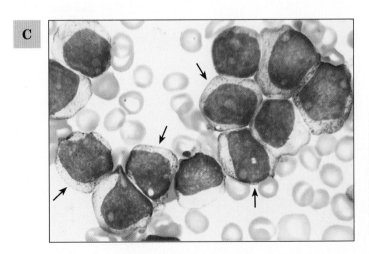

Blood smear. (Courtesy Dr Robert W. McKenna, Department of Pathology, University of Texas Southwestern Medical School, Dallas, Texas; from Kumar V, Cotran RS, Robbins SL: *Basic Pathology,* ed 7, Philadelphia, 2003, WB Saunders.)

1. In this blood smear, the arrows point to an increased number of large, immature cells (that would normally fight infection). They are:

a. hepatocytes
b. erythrocytes
c. thrombocytes
d. leukocytes

2. The name of the abnormal condition in which these cells predominate is:

a. iron deficiency anemia
b. sickle-cell anemia
c. leukemia
d. hyperglycemia

Answers to Picture Show

A

1. c   2. d   3. a

B

1. b

C

1. d   2. c

VIII. Medical Scramble

Unscramble the letters to form a medical term from the clues. Use the letters in squares to complete the bonus term. Answers are upside down at the bottom of the page.

1. Pertaining to the heart

   C A R D I A C DACCIRA

2. Nerve pain

   N E U R A L G I A UGARENLAI

3. Deficiency of hemoglobin causes this condition

   ___ ___ ___ [ ] ___ ___ IMEANA

4. Study of cells

   [ ] ___ ___ ___ ___ [ ] ___ ___ GLYCOTOY

5. Infants are often born in this position...head first!

   [ ] ___ ___ ___ ___ ___ [ ] ___ PCLAHIEC

6. Inflammation of a gland

   [ ] ___ ___ [ ] ___ ___ ___ ___ NIDIEAST

BONUS TERM: MALIGNANT DIAGNOSIS

[ ] [ ] [ ] [ ] [ ] [ ] [ ] [ ] [ ]

2

Organization of the Body

Chapter Sections

Chapter Objectives

- To name the body systems and their functions
- To identify body cavities and specific organs within them
- To list the divisions of the back
- To identify three planes of the body
- To analyze, pronounce, and spell new terms related to organs and tissues in the body

I. Body Systems

All the parts of your body are composed of individual units called **cells.** Muscle, nerve, skin (epithelial), and bone cells are examples.

Similar cells grouped together are **tissues.** Groups of muscle cells are muscle tissue, and groups of epithelial cells are epithelial tissue.

Collections of different tissues working together are **organs.** An organ, such as the stomach, has different tissues, such as muscle, epithelial (lining of internal organs and outer layer of skin cells), and nerve, that help the organ function.

Groups of organs working together are the **systems** of the body. The digestive system, for example, includes organs such as the mouth, throat, esophagus, stomach, and intestines that bring food into the body and deliver it to the bloodstream.

There are 11 systems of the body, and each plays an important role in the way the body works.

The **circulatory system** (heart, blood, and blood vessels such as arteries, veins, and capillaries) transports blood throughout the body. The **lymphatic system** includes lymph vessels and nodes that carry a clear fluid called lymph. Lymph contains white blood cells called lymphocytes that fight against disease and play an important role in immunity.

The **digestive system** brings food into the body and breaks it down so that it can enter the bloodstream. Food that cannot be broken down is then removed from the body at the end of the system.

The **endocrine system,** composed of glands, sends chemical messengers called hormones into the blood to act on other glands and organs.

The **female and male reproductive systems** produce the cells that join to form the embryo. Male (testis) and female (ovary) sex organs produce hormones as well.

The **musculoskeletal system,** including muscles, bones, joints, and connective tissues, supports the body and allows it to move.

The **nervous system** carries electrical messages to and from the brain and spinal cord.

The **respiratory system** controls breathing, a process in which air enters and leaves the body.

The **skin and sense organ system,** including the skin and eyes and ears, receives messages from the environment and sends them to the brain.

The **urinary system** produces urine and sends it out of the body through the kidneys, ureters, bladder, and urethra.

Appendix I, at the back of the book, contains diagrams of each body system with combining forms for body parts, examples of terminology, pathology, and laboratory tests, and diagnostic and treatment procedures. *Appendix II* names and explains common diagnostic tests and procedures, and *Appendix III* defines medical abbreviations, acronyms, and symbols. Two glossaries, the *Glossary of Medical Terms,* p. 313, and *Glossary of Word Parts,* p. 347, contain definitions of terms and meanings of word parts. Use these appendices and glossaries as references during your study and later as you work in the medical field.

II. Body Cavities

Figure 2-1 shows the five body cavities. A body cavity is a space that contains organs. Label Figure 2-1 as you read the following paragraphs.

The **cranial cavity** (1) is located in the head and is surrounded by the skull (CRANI/O means skull). The brain and other organs, such as the pituitary gland (an endocrine gland below the brain), are in the cranial cavity.

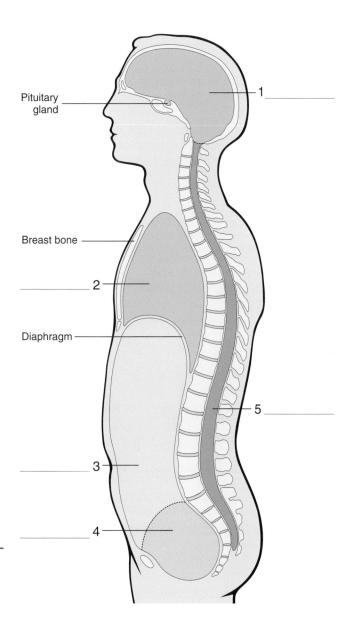

Pituitary gland

Breast bone

Diaphragm

FIGURE 2–1

Body cavities. (Modified from Chabner D-E: *The Language of Medicine,* ed 7, Philadelphia, 2004, WB Saunders.)

The **thoracic cavity** (2) is the chest cavity (THORAC/O means chest), which is surrounded by the breastbone and ribs. The lungs, heart, windpipe (trachea), bronchial tubes (leading from the trachea to the lungs), and other organs are in the thoracic cavity.

Figure 2-2 shows a front view of the thoracic cavity. The lungs are each surrounded by a double membrane known as the **pleura.** The space between the pleura and surrounding each lung is the **pleural cavity.** The large space between the lungs is the **mediastinum.** The heart, esophagus (food tube), trachea, and bronchial tubes are organs within the mediastinum.

In Figure 2-1, the **abdominal cavity** (3) is the space below the thoracic cavity. The **diaphragm** is the muscle that separates the abdominal and thoracic cavities. Organs in the abdomen include the stomach, liver, gallbladder, and small and large intestines.

The organs in the abdomen are covered by a membrane called the **peritoneum** (Figure 2-3). The peritoneum attaches the abdominal organs to the abdominal muscles and surrounds each organ to hold it in place.

Turn back to Figure 2-1 and locate the **pelvic cavity** (4), below the abdominal cavity. The pelvic cavity is surrounded by the **pelvis** (bones of the hip). The organs located within the pelvic cavity are the urinary bladder, ureters (tubes from the

FIGURE 2–2

Thoracic cavity.

Lung

Peritoneum

Liver

Stomach

Kidney

Large intestine

Retroperitoneal area

Omentum (part of the peritoneum)

Small intestine

Uterus

Urinary bladder

Rectum

Urethra

Anus

Vagina

FIGURE 2–3

The **peritoneum** surrounds the organs in the abdomen.

kidneys to the bladder), urethra (tube from the bladder to the outside of the body), rectum and anus, and the uterus (muscular organ that nourishes the developing embryo and fetus) in females.

Figure 2-1 on p. 45 also shows the **spinal cavity** (5). This is the space surrounded by the **spinal column** (backbones). The **spinal cord** is the nervous tissue within the spinal cavity. Nerves enter and leave the spinal cord and carry messages to and from all parts of the body.

As a quick review of the terms presented in this section, match the term with its meaning and write it on the space provided.

Term	Meaning

Abdominal cavity

Cranial cavity

Diaphragm

Mediastinum

Pelvic cavity

Pelvis

Peritoneum

Pleura

Spinal cavity

Thoracic cavity

1. Membrane surrounding the lungs _____

2. Space between the lungs, containing the heart

   _____

3. Bones of the hip _____

4. Space containing the liver, gallbladder, and stomach; also

   called the abdomen _____

5. Space within the backbones, containing the spinal cord

   _____

6. Membrane surrounding the organs in the abdomen

   _____

7. Space within the skull, containing the brain

   _____

8. Space below the abdominal cavity, containing the urinary

   bladder _____

9. Muscle between the thoracic and abdominal cavities

   _____

10. Entire chest cavity, containing the lungs, heart, trachea,

    esophagus, and bronchial tubes _____

III. Divisions of the Back

The **spinal column** is a long row of bones from the neck to the tailbone. Each bone in the spinal column is called a **vertebra** (backbone). Two or more bones are **vertebrae.**

A piece of flexible connective tissue, called a **disk** (or **disc**), lies between each backbone. The disk, composed of **cartilage,** is a cushion between the bones. If the disk slips, or moves out of its place, it can press on the nerves that enter or leave the spinal cord and cause pain. Figure 2-4 shows a side view of vertebrae and disks.

The divisions of the spinal column are pictured in Figure 2-5. Label them according to the following list:

Division	Bones	Abbreviation
1. **Cervical** (neck) region	7 bones	C1-C7
2. **Thoracic** (chest) region	12 bones	T1-T12
3. **Lumbar** (loin or waist) region	5 bones	L1-L5
4. **Sacral** (sacrum or lower back) region	5 fused bones	S1-S5
5. **Coccygeal** (coccyx or tailbone) region	4 fused bones	

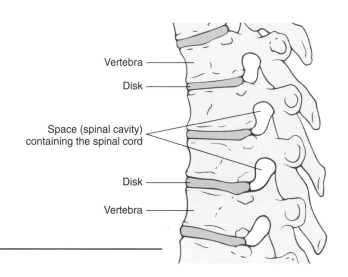

FIGURE 2–4

Vertebrae and disks (discs).

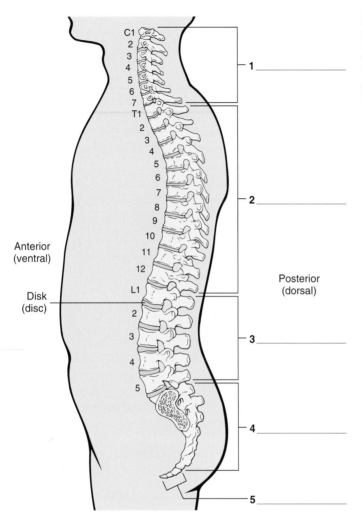

Anterior
(ventral)

Disk
(disc)

Posterior
(dorsal)

C1
2
3
4
5
6
7
T1
2
3
4
5
6
7
8
9
10
11
12
L1
2
3
4
5

1 _____

2 _____

3 _____

4 _____

5 _____

FIGURE 2–5

Divisions of the back (spinal column). (Modified from Chabner D-E: *The Language of Medicine,* ed 7, Philadelphia, 2004, WB Saunders.)

IV. Planes of the Body

A plane is an imaginary flat surface. Organs appear in different relationships to each other according to the plane of the body in which they are viewed.

Figure 2-6 shows three planes of the body. Label them as you read the following descriptions:

1. **Frontal (coronal) plane**   An up-and-down plane that divides the body or an organ into front (**anterior,** or **A**) and back (**posterior,** or **P**) portions. A routine chest x-ray (A/P or P/A) film shows the thoracic cavity in the frontal plane. See Figure 2-7, *A.*

FIGURE 2–6

Planes of the body.

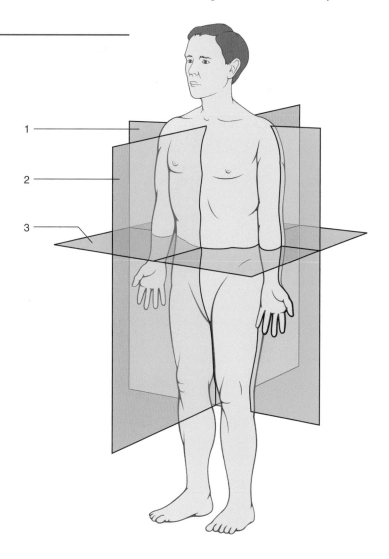

1

2

3

2. **Sagittal (lateral) plane**   A plane that divides the body or an organ into a right and left side. A lateral chest x-ray (see Figure 2-7, *B*) shows the thoracic cavity in the sagittal, or lateral, plane.

3. **Transverse (axial) plane**   A plane that divides the body or an organ into upper and lower portions, as in a **cross-section.** A **CT scan** is an x-ray image of the body taken in the transverse (axial) plane. Figure 2-7, *C,* is a CT scan of the chest.

A

Lung
Ribs
Heart

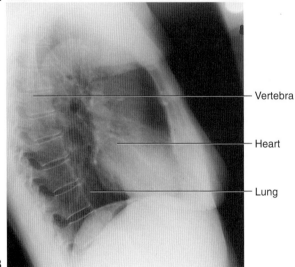

B

Vertebra
Heart
Lung

FIGURE 2–7

X-ray views of the chest.
A, Frontal, or coronal, plane;
B, sagittal, or lateral, plane;
and **C,** transverse, or axial,
plane. (**A,** Modified from Black
JM, Matassarin-Jacobs E:
*Medical-Surgical Nursing:
Clinical Management for
Continuity of Care,* ed 5,
Philadelphia, 1997, WB
Saunders. **B,** Modified from
Weir J, Abrahams PH: *An
Imaging Atlas of Human
Anatomy,* ed 2, London, 2000,
Mosby. **C,** From Chabner D-E:
The Language of Medicine,
ed 7, Philadelphia, 2004,
WB Saunders.)

Right
Left

Lungs
Bone of rib
Vertebra

C

Magnetic resonance imaging (MRI) is another technique for producing images of the body. Instead of x-rays, MRI creates images using magnetic waves. The images from MRI show organs in all three planes (frontal, sagittal, and transverse) of the body (Figure 2-8). Figure 2-9 shows a patient undergoing MRI.

A   B

C

FIGURE 2–8

Magnetic resonance images. A, Frontal (coronal) view of the upper body. White masses in the chest are tumors. **B,** Transverse (axial) view of the same patient with chest mass. **C,** Sagittal (lateral) view of the brain. (**A** and **B,** From Chabner D-E: *The Language of Medicine,* ed 7, Philadelphia, 2004, WB Saunders. **C,** Modified from Black JM, Matassarin-Jacobs E: *Medical-Surgical Nursing: Clinical Management for Continuity of Care,* ed 5, Philadelphia, 1997, WB Saunders.)

FIGURE 2–9

Patient is inside an MRI unit, surrounded by a superconducting 1.5-tesla magnet. Magnetic field changes are picked up by the surrounding machine and processed by a computer to create images. Patients must lie very still and have no metal objects on or within their body. (Courtesy GE Medical Systems, Milwaukee, Wisconsin. In Ballinger PW, Frank ED: *Merrill's Atlas of Radiographic Positions and Radiologic Procedures,* ed 10, St Louis, 2003, Mosby.)

V. Terminology

Write the meanings of the medical terms on the line provided. Check your answers with the *Glossary of Medical Terms,* p. 313.

Combining Forms

Combining Form	Meaning	Medical Term	Meaning
abdomin/o	abdomen	abdominal _____	
anter/o	front	anterior _____ *The suffix* -IOR *means pertaining to.*	
bronch/o	bronchial tubes (leading from the windpipe to the lungs)	bronchoscopy _____	
cervic/o	*neck* of the body or *neck* (cervix) of the uterus	cervical _____ *You must decide from the context of what you are reading whether* **cervical** *means pertaining to the neck of the body or pertaining to the cervix (lower portion or the uterus). Figure 2-10 shows the uterus and the cervix.*	

FIGURE 2–10

The uterus and cervix.

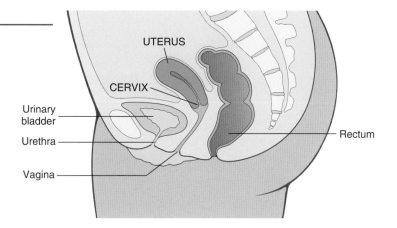

UTERUS

CERVIX

Urinary bladder

Urethra

Vagina

Rectum

chondr/o	cartilage	hypochondriac _____
		This term refers to the regions of the abdominopelvic cavity under the cartilage of the ribs. See Figure A (abdominopelvic regions), p. 72. It also describes a person with unusual anxiety about health and with symptoms that cannot be explained. The Greeks thought organs (liver and spleen) in the hypochondriac regions of the abdomen were the origin of imaginary illnesses.
coccyg/o	coccyx, tailbone	coccygeal _____
		-EAL means pertaining to.
crani/o	skull	craniotomy _____
epitheli/o	skin, surface tissue	epithelial _____
		*The term **epithelial** was first used to describe the surface (EPI- means upon) of the breast nipple (THELI/O means nipple). Currently, it describes the cells on the outer layer (surface) of the skin as well as the lining of the internal organs that lead to the outside of the body.*
esophag/o	esophagus (tube from the throat to the stomach)	esophageal _____
hepat/o	liver	hepatitis _____
lapar/o	abdomen	laparoscopy _____

2

laryng/o	larynx (voice box)	laryngeal _____

The larynx (pronounced **LAR**-*inks) is found in the upper part of the trachea.*

laryngectomy _____

later/o	side	lateral _____
lumb/o	loin (waist)	lumbar _____

-AR *means pertaining to. A lumbar puncture is the placement of a needle within the membranes in the lumbar region of the spinal cord to inject or withdraw fluid. See Figure 2-11.*

lymph/o	lymph (clear fluid in tissue spaces and lymph vessels)	lymphocyte _____

Lymphocytes are white blood cells and are important in fighting disease. They produce disease-fighting proteins called **antibodies.**

mediastin/o	mediastinum (space between the lungs)	mediastinal _____
pelv/o	pelvis (bones of the hip)	pelvic _____

FIGURE 2–11

Lumbar (spinal) puncture. The patient lies laterally, with the knees drawn up to the abdomen and the chin brought down to the chest. This position increases the spaces between the vertebrae. The lumbar puncture needle is inserted between the third and fourth (or fourth and fifth) lumbar vertebrae, and fluid can be injected or withdrawn. The distal end of the spinal cord is where the spinal nerves begin to fan out toward the legs. The lumbar puncture is performed below this area to avoid injury to the spinal cord. (Modified from Chabner D-E: *The Language of Medicine,* ed 7, Philadelphia, 2004, WB Saunders.)

FIGURE 2–12

Pharynx. Notice that the epiglottis (a flap of cartilage) closes over the trachea during swallowing so that the bolus of food travels down the esophagus. (Modified from Chabner D-E: *The Language of Medicine,* ed 7, Philadelphia, 2004, WB Saunders.)

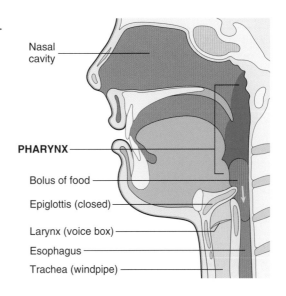

Nasal cavity

PHARYNX

Bolus of food

Epiglottis (closed)

Larynx (voice box)

Esophagus

Trachea (windpipe)

peritone/o	peritoneum (membrane surrounding the abdomen)	peritoneal _____
pharyng/o	pharynx (throat)	pharyngeal _____

The pharynx (pronounced **FAR***-inks) is the common passageway for food from the mouth and air from the nose. See Figure 2-12.*

pleur/o	pleura	pleuritis _____
poster/o	back, behind	posterior _____
sacr/o	sacrum (five fused bones in the lower back)	sacral _____
spin/o	spine (backbone)	spinal _____
thorac/o	chest	thoracotomy _____
		thoracic _____

FIGURE 2–13

Tracheotomy.

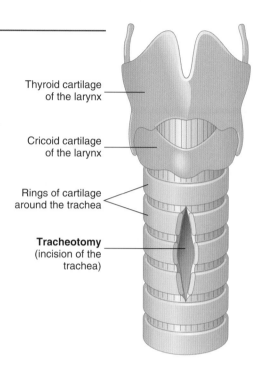

Thyroid cartilage
of the larynx

Cricoid cartilage
of the larynx

Rings of cartilage
around the trachea

Tracheotomy
(incision of the
trachea)

trache/o	trachea (windpipe)	tracheotomy _____
		See Figure 2-13.
vertebr/o	vertebra (backbone)	vertebral _____

VI. Exercises and Answers

Complete these exercises and check your answers. An important part of your success in learning medical terminology is checking your answers carefully with the answer key beginning on p. 64.

A. Match the following systems of the body with their functions.

circulatory	musculoskeletal	respiratory
digestive	nervous	skin and sense organs
endocrine	reproductive	urinary

1. Produces urine and sends it out of the body: _____

2. Secretes hormones that are carried by blood to other organs: _____

3. Supports the body and helps it move: _____

4. Takes food into the body; breaks it down so it is absorbed into the bloodstream:

_____

5. Transports food, gases, and other substances through the body: _____

_____

6. Moves air in and out of the body: _____

7. Produces the cells that unite to form a new baby: _____

8. Receives messages from the environment and sends them to the brain: _____

_____

9. Carries electrical messages to and from the brain and spinal cord: _____

_____

B. Use the following terms to complete the chart below. Give the name of the cavity and an organ that is contained within the cavity.

abdominal	lungs	stomach
brain	pelvic	thoracic
cranial	spinal	urinary bladder
heart	spinal cord	uterus

	Cavity	Organ
1. Space contained within the bones of the hip	_____	_____
2. Space contained within the skull	_____	_____
3. Space contained within the chest	_____	_____
4. Space contained within the abdomen	_____	_____
5. Space contained within the backbones	_____	_____

C. Complete the following sentences using the terms listed below.

abdomen (abdominal cavity)	mediastinum	spinal column
diaphragm	pelvis	spinal cord
disk (disc)	peritoneum	vertebra
	pleura	

1. The bones of the hip are the _____.

2. The muscle separating the chest and the abdomen is the _____.

3. The membrane surrounding the organs in the abdomen is the _____.

4. The membrane surrounding the lungs is the _____.

5. The space between the lungs in the chest is the _____.

6. The space that contains organs such as the stomach, liver, gallbladder, and

   intestines is the _____.

7. The backbones are the _____.

8. The nerves running down the back form the _____.

9. A single backbone is a _____.

10. A piece of cartilage in between each backbone is a _____.

D. Name the five divisions of the spinal column from the neck to the tailbone.

1. C __ __ __ __ __ __ __

2. T __ __ __ __ __ __ __

3. L __ __ __ __ __

4. S __ __ __ __ __

5. C __ __ __ __ __ __ __ __

E. Match the following terms with their meanings below.

anterior frontal (coronal) plane sagittal plane
cartilage MRI transverse (axial) plane
CT scan posterior

1. Pertaining to the back: _____

2. Pertaining to the front: _____

3. A plane that divides the body into an upper and lower part: _____

4. An image of the body using magnetic waves; all three planes of the body are

    viewed: _____

5. A plane that divides the body into right and left parts: _____

6. Flexible connective tissue found between bones at joints: _____

7. A plane that divides the body into front and back parts: _____

8. Series of cross-sectional x-ray images: _____

F. Give meanings for the following terms.

1. craniotomy _____

2. abdominal _____

3. pelvic _____

4. thoracic _____

5. mediastinal _____

6. epithelial _____

7. tracheotomy _____

8. peritoneal _____

9. hepatitis _____

10. cervical _____

11. lymphocyte _____

12. lateral _____

13. bronchoscopy _____

14. diaphragm _____

15. pleura _____

16. hypochondriac _____

G. Match the following terms with their meanings below.

coccygeal	laparotomy	pleuritis
epithelial	laryngeal	sacral
esophageal	lumbar	thoracotomy
laparoscopy	pharyngeal	vertebral

1. Pertaining to the loin (waist) region under the thoracic vertebrae: _____

2. Pertaining to skin (lining or surface) cells: _____

3. Incision of the abdomen: _____

4. Pertaining to the tube from the throat to stomach: _____

5. Pertaining to the voice box: _____

6. Inflammation of the membrane surrounding the lungs: _____

7. Pertaining to the throat: _____

8. Pertaining to the sacrum: _____

9. Incision of the chest: _____

10. Pertaining to the tailbone: _____

11. Visual examination of the abdomen: _____

12. Pertaining to backbones: _____

H. Circle the term that best completes the meaning of the sentences in the following medical vignettes.

1. After her car accident, Cathy had severe neck pain. An MRI revealed a protruding **(diaphragm, disk, uterus)** between C6 and C7. The doctor asked her to wear a **(sacral, cervical, cranial)** collar for several weeks.

2. Mr. Sellar was a heavy smoker all his adult life. He began coughing and losing weight and became very lethargic (tired). His physician suspected a tumor of the **(musculoskeletal, urinary, respiratory)** system. A chest CT showed a **(lung, pharyngeal, spinal)** mass. Dr. Baker performed **(laparoscopy, craniotomy, bronchoscopy)** to biopsy the lesion.

3. Grace had never seen a gynecologist. She had pain in her **(cranial, pelvic, thoracic)** cavity and increasing **(abdominal, vertebral, laryngeal)** girth (size). Dr. Hawk suspected a(an) **(esophageal, ovarian, mediastinal)** tumor after palpating (examining by touch) a mass.

4. Mr. Cruise worked in the shipyards for several years during World War II. Now, many years later, his doctor encouraged him to stop smoking because of a recently discovered link between asbestos, smoking, and the occurrence of mesothelioma (malignant tumor of cells of the pleura or the membrane surrounding the lungs). On a routine chest x-ray, there had been thickening of the **(esophagus, pleura, trachea)** on both sides of Mr. Cruise's **(abdominal, spinal, thoracic)** cavity.

5. Kelly complained of headaches, together with nausea, disturbances of vision, and loss of coordination in her movements. Also, she had weakness, and stiffness on one side of her body. Dr. Brown suspected a tumor of the central **(circulatory, digestive, nervous)** system. Treatment involved a **(thoracotomy, craniotomy, laryngectomy)** to remove the lesion (mass) in her brain.

6. Mr. Jones experienced increasing weakness and loss of movement in his left arm and left leg. He saw his family doctor, who immediately referred him to a **(neurologist, cardiologist, rheumatologist)**. This specialist examined him and sent him to **(pathology, hematology, radiology)** for x-ray imaging. (Results are shown in Figure 2-14.) This image is a(an) **(MRI, CT scan, A/P film)**. The imaging clearly showed a large white region in the brain, indicating an area of dead tissue. Mr. Jones' doctor informed him that he had had a stroke, which is also known as a **(pituitary gland tumor, myocardial infarction, CVA or cerebrovascular accident)**.

2

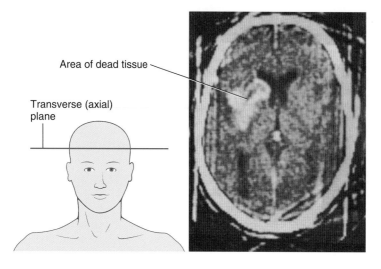

Area of dead tissue

Transverse (axial) plane

FIGURE 2–14

Cross-sectional x-ray image of Mr. Smith's head.

Answers to Exercises

A

1. urinary
2. endocrine
3. musculoskeletal
4. digestive
5. circulatory
6. respiratory
7. reproductive
8. skin and sense organs
9. nervous

B

1. pelvic (urinary bladder, uterus)
2. cranial (brain)
3. thoracic (lungs, heart)
4. abdominal (stomach)
5. spinal (spinal cord)

C

1. pelvis
2. diaphragm
3. peritoneum
4. pleura
5. mediastinum
6. abdomen (abdominal cavity)
7. spinal column
8. spinal cord
9. vertebra
10. disk (disc)

D

1. cervical
2. thoracic
3. lumbar
4. sacral
5. coccygeal

E

1. posterior
2. anterior
3. transverse (axial) plane
4. MRI
5. sagittal plane
6. cartilage
7. frontal (coronal) plane
8. CT scan

F

1. incision of the skull
2. pertaining to the abdomen
3. pertaining to the pelvis (bones of the hip)
4. pertaining to the chest
5. pertaining to the mediastinum (the space between the lungs)
6. pertaining to skin (lining or surface) cells
7. incision of the trachea (windpipe)
8. pertaining to the peritoneum (the membrane surrounding the organs in the abdomen)
9. inflammation of the liver
10. pertaining to the neck of the body, or neck (cervix) of the uterus
11. lymph cell (a type of white blood cell)
12. pertaining to the side
13. visual examination of bronchial tubes using an endoscope
14. muscle separating the abdomen from the chest
15. membrane surrounding the lungs
16. pertaining to under the cartilage of the rib (two upper lateral areas of the abdomen); or describing a person with unusual anxiety about symptoms that cannot be explained

G

1. lumbar	5. laryngeal	9. thoracotomy
2. epithelial	6. pleuritis	10. coccygeal
3. laparotomy	7. pharyngeal	11. laparoscopy
4. esophageal	8. sacral	12. vertebral

H

1. disk, cervical	4. pleura, thoracic
2. respiratory, lung, bronchoscopy	5. nervous, craniotomy
3. pelvic, abdominal, ovarian	6. neurologist, radiology, CT scan, CVA or cerebrovascular accident

VII. Review

Write the meanings of the following combining forms and suffixes in the spaces provided. Check your answers with the answer key at the end of the section on p. 67. Meanings for word parts are also listed in the *Glossary of Word Parts* beginning on p. 347.

Combining Forms

Combining Form	Meaning	Combining Form	Meaning
1. abdomin/o _____		3. bronch/o _____	
2. anter/o _____		4. cervic/o _____	

5. chondr/o _____

6. coccyg/o _____

7. crani/o _____

8. epitheli/o _____

9. esophag/o _____

10. hepat/o _____

11. lapar/o _____

12. laryng/o _____

13. later/o _____

14. lumb/o _____

15. lymph/o _____

16. mediastin/o _____

17. pelv/o _____

18. peritone/o _____

19. pharyng/o _____

20. pleur/o _____

21. poster/o _____

22. sacr/o _____

23. spin/o _____

24. thorac/o _____

25. trache/o _____

26. vertebr/o _____

Suffixes

Suffix	Meaning	Suffix	Meaning
1. -ac		7. -ic	
2. -al		8. -itis	
3. -ar		9. -logy	
4. -cyte		10. -oma	
5. -eal		11. -scopy	
6. -ectomy		12. -tomy	

Answers to Review

Combining Forms

1. abdomen	10. liver	19. throat
2. front	11. abdomen	20. pleura
3. bronchial tubes	12. voice box	21. back, behind
4. neck	13. side	22. sacrum
5. cartilage	14. loin, waist region	23. backbone
6. tailbone	15. lymph	24. chest
7. skull	16. mediastinum	25. windpipe
8. skin	17. bones of the hip region	26. backbone
9. esophagus	18. peritoneum	

Suffixes

1. pertaining to	6. removal, excision, resection	9. study of
2. pertaining to		10. tumor, mass
3. pertaining to	7. pertaining to	11. process of viewing
4. cell	8. inflammation	12. incision, to cut into
5. pertaining to		

VIII. Pronunciation of Terms

The terms that you have learned in this chapter are presented here with their pronunciations. The capitalized letters in boldface represent the accented syllable. Pronounce each word out loud, then write the meaning in the space provided. Meanings of terms are found in the *Glossary of Medical Terms*, p. 313.

Term	Pronunciation	Meaning
abdomen	**AB**-do-men	
abdominal cavity	ab-**DOM**-in-al **KAV**-i-te	
anterior	an-**TE**-re-or	
bronchial tubes	**BRONG**-ke-al tubes	
bronchoscopy	bron-**KOS**-ko-pe	
cartilage	**KAR**-tih-lij	
cervical	**SER**-vi-kal	

circulatory system	**SER**-ku-lah-tor-e **SIS**-tem	_____
coccygeal	kok-sih-**JE**-al	_____
coccyx	**KOK**-siks	_____
cranial cavity	**KRA**-ne-al **KAV**-ih-te	_____
craniotomy	kra-ne-**OT**-o-me	_____
diaphragm	**DI**-ah-fram	_____
digestive system	di-**JES**-tiv **SIS**-tem	_____
disk (disc)	disk	_____
endocrine system	**EN**-do-krin **SIS**-tem	_____
epithelial	ep-ih-**THE**-le-al	_____
esophageal	eh-sof-ah-**JE**-al	_____
esophagus	eh-**SOF**-ah-gus	_____
female reproductive system	**FE**-mal re-pro-**DUK**-tiv **SIS**-tem	_____
frontal plane	**FRUN**-tal plan	_____
hepatitis	hep-ah-**TI**-tis	_____
hypochondriac	hi-po-**KON**-dre-ak	_____
laparoscopy	lap-ah-**ROS**-ko-pe	_____
laparotomy	lap-ah-**ROT**-o-me	_____
laryngeal	lah-**RIN**-je-al or lah-rin-**JE**-al	_____
laryngectomy	lah-rin-**JEK**-to-me	_____
larynx	**LAR**-inks	_____
lateral	**LAT**-er-al	_____
lumbar	**LUM**-bar	_____

lymphocyte	**LIMF**-o-site _____
mediastinal	me-de-as-**TI**-nal _____
mediastinum	me-de-ahs-**TI**-num _____
musculoskeletal system	mus-ku-lo-**SKEL**-e-tal **SIS**-tem _____
nervous system	**NER**-vus **SIS**-tem _____
ovary	**O**-vah-re _____
pelvic cavity	**PEL**-vik **KAV**-ih-te _____
pelvis	**PEL**-vis _____
peritoneal	per-ih-to-**NE**-al _____
peritoneum	per-ih-to-**NE**-um _____
pharyngeal	fah-**RIN**-je-al or fah-rin-**JE**-al _____
pharynx	**FAR**-inks _____
pituitary gland	pih-**TU**-ih-tah-re gland _____
pleura	**PLOO**-rah _____
pleuritis	ploo-**RI**-tis _____
posterior	pos-**TER**-e-or _____
respiratory system	**RES**-pir-ah-tor-e **SIS**-tem _____
sacral	**SA**-kral _____
sacrum	**SA**-krum _____
sagittal plane	**SAJ**-ih-tal plan _____
spinal cavity	**SPI**-nal **KAV**-ih-te _____
spinal column	**SPI**-nal **KOL**-um _____
spinal cord	**SPI**-nal kord _____

thoracic cavity   tho-**RAS**-ik **KAV**-ih-te _____

thoracotomy   tho-rah-**KOT**-o-me _____

trachea   **TRAY**-ke-ah _____

tracheotomy   tray-ke-**OT**-o-me _____

transverse plane   trans-**VERS** plan _____

ureter   **YOOR**-eh-ter or u-**RE**-ter _____

urethra   u-**RE**-thrah _____

urinary system   **UR**-in-er-e **SIS**-tem _____

uterus   **U**-ter-us _____

vertebra   **VER**-teh-brah _____

vertebrae   **VER**-teh-bray _____

vertebral   **VER**-teh-bral _____

IX. **Practical Applications**

Select one of the procedures listed below to identify the descriptions in the following paragraphs. Answers are found on p. 71.

bronchoscopy   laparotomy   thoracotomy
craniotomy   laryngectomy   tracheotomy
laparoscopy

1. A skin incision is made, and muscle is stripped away from the skull. Four or five

   burr (bur) holes are drilled into the skull. The bone between the holes is cut using

   a craniotome (bone saw). The bone flap is turned down or completely removed.

   After the bone flap is secured, the membrane surrounding the brain is incised and

   the brain is exposed. This procedure is a _____.

2. A major surgical incision is made into the chest for diagnostic or therapeutic purposes. One type of incision is a medial sternotomy (the sternum is the breast bone). A straight incision is made from the upper part of the sternum (suprasternal notch) to the lower end of the sternum (xiphoid process). The sternum must be cut with an electric or air-driven saw. The procedure is done to perform a biopsy or to locate sources of bleeding or injury. It is often performed to remove all or a portion of the lung. This procedure is a _____.

3. A needle is inserted below the umbilicus (navel) to infuse carbon dioxide (a gas) into the abdomen. This distends (expands) the abdomen and permits better visualization of the organs. A trocar (sharp-pointed instrument used to puncture the wall of a body cavity) within a cannula (tube) is inserted into an incision under the umbilicus. After it is in place in the abdominal cavity, the trocar is removed and an endoscope is inserted through the cannula. The surgeon can thus visualize the abdominopelvic cavity and reproductive organs. This procedure is a _____.

4. A flexible, fiberoptic endoscope is inserted through the mouth, throat, and trachea to assess the tracheobronchial tree for tumors and obstructions, to perform biopsies, and to remove secretions and foreign bodies. This procedure is a _____.

Answers to Practical Applications

1. craniotomy
2. thoracotomy
3. laparoscopy
4. bronchoscopy

X. Picture Show

Answer the questions that follow each image. Correct answers are on p. 74.

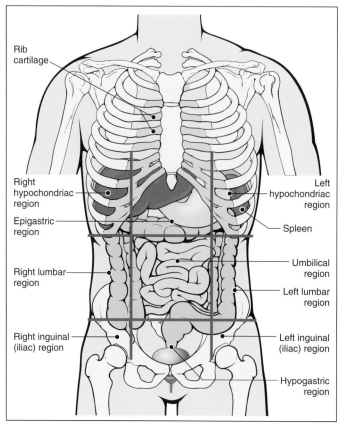

Abdominopelvic regions. (Modified from Chabner D-E: *The Language of Medicine,* ed 7, Philadelphia, 2004, WB Saunders.)

1. Which abdominopelvic regions are the middle lateral regions?

    a. epigastric   c. hypochondriac
    b. lumbar   d. inguinal

2. Which abdominopelvic region lies above the stomach?

    a. epigastric   c. umbilical
    b. inguinal   d. hypogastric

3. Which abdominopelvic regions lie under the cartilage of the ribs?

    a. hypogastric   c. umbilical
    b. hypochondriac   d. inguinal

4. Which lateral abdominopelvic regions are in the area of the groin (depression between the thigh and the trunk of the body)?

     a. umbilical   c. lumbar
     b. hypochondriac   d. inguinal

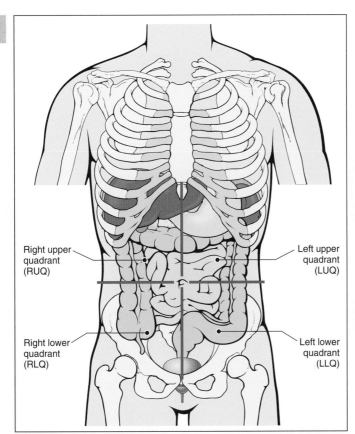

Abdominopelvic quadrants. (Modified from Chabner D-E: *The Language of Medicine,* ed 7, Philadelphia, 2004, WB Saunders.)

1. A large organ in the RUQ is the

     a. stomach   c. heart
     b. lung   d. liver

2. The spleen is located in which quadrant?

     a. LUQ   c. RLQ
     b. RUQ   d. LLQ

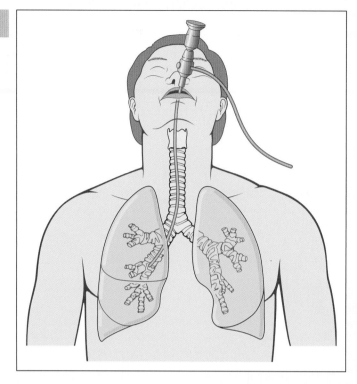

C

1. In the image, an endoscope is inserted into the mouth to visualize tubes leading to the lungs. This procedure is:

   a. laryngoscopy
   b. laparoscopy
   c. mediastinoscopy
   d. esophagoscopy
   e. bronchoscopy

Answers to Picture Show

A

1. b   2. a   3. b   4. d

B

1. d   2. a

C

1. e. This procedure is used for removing material (sputum) from the bronchial tubes, obtaining a biopsy specimen, or removing foreign bodies.

XI. Medical Scramble

Unscramble the letters to form a medical term from the clues. Use the letters in squares to complete the bonus term. Answers are upside down at the bottom of the page.

1. Female endocrine organ

   ☐ __ __ __ ☐   R O A Y V

2. Space below the diaphragm

   ☐ __ __ __ ☐ __ __   E B M A O N D

3. Pertaining to the chest

   __ __ ☐ __ __ ☐ __ __   H C I R A O C T

4. Bones of the hip

   __ __ __ __ ☐ __   L E P V S I

5. Throat

   __ __ __ ☐ __ ☐ __   R P Y X N A H

6. Windpipe

   ☐ __ __ __ __ __ __   A C E T H R A

   BONUS TERM: A PROCEDURE NECESSARY FOR BRAIN SURGERY

   ☐ ☐ ☐ ☐ ☐ ☐ ☐ ☐ ☐ ☐

3

Suffixes

Chapter Sections

Chapter Objectives

- To identify and define useful diagnostic and procedural suffixes
- To analyze, spell, and pronounce medical terms that contain diagnostic and procedural suffixes

I. Introduction

This chapter reviews the suffixes that you have learned in the first two chapters and also introduces new suffixes and medical terms. The combining forms used in the chapter are listed below in Section II. Refer to this list as you write the meanings of the terms in Section III. Be faithful about completing all exercises in Section IV, and remember to check your answers on p. 103! These exercises will help you spell terms correctly and understand their meanings. Test yourself by completing the Review in Section V and Pronunciation of Terms in Section VI.

II. Combining Forms

Combining Form	Meaning
aden/o	gland
amni/o	amnion (sac of fluid surrounding the embryo)
angi/o	vessel (usually a blood vessel)
arteri/o	artery
arthr/o	joint
ather/o	plaque (a yellow, fatty material)
axill/o	armpit (underarm)
bronch/o	bronchial tube
bronchi/o	bronchial tube
carcin/o	cancerous
cardi/o	heart
chem/o	drug (or chemical)
cholecyst/o	gallbladder
chron/o	time
col/o	colon (large intestine or bowel)
crani/o	skull
cry/o	cold
cyst/o	urinary bladder; also a sac of fluid or cyst
electr/o	electricity
encephal/o	brain
erythr/o	red
esophag/o	esophagus (tube leading from the throat to the stomach)
hem/o	blood
hemat/o	blood
hepat/o	liver
hyster/o	uterus
inguin/o	groin (area where the thigh meets the trunk of the body)
isch/o	to hold back
lapar/o	abdomen (abdominal wall)

laryng/o	voice box (larynx)
leuk/o	white
mamm/o	breast (use with -ARY, -GRAPHY, -GRAM, and -PLASTY)
mast/o	breast (use with -ECTOMY and -ITIS)
men/o	menses (menstruation); month
mening/o	meninges (membranes around the brain and spinal cord)
my/o	muscle
myel/o	spinal cord (nervous tissue connected to the brain and located within the spinal column or backbone); in other terms, MYEL/O- means bone marrow (the soft, inner part of bones, where blood cells are made)
necr/o	death (of cells)
nephr/o	kidney (use with all suffixes, except -AL and -GRAM; use REN/O with -AL and -GRAM)
neur/o	nerve
oophor/o	ovary
oste/o	bone
ot/o	ear
pelv/o	hip area
peritone/o	peritoneum (membrane surrounding the organs in the abdominal cavity)
phleb/o	vein
pneumon/o	lung
pulmon/o	lung
radi/o	x-rays
ren/o	kidney (use with -AL and -GRAM)
rhin/o	nose
salping/o	fallopian (uterine) tube
sarc/o	flesh
septic/o	pertaining to infection
thorac/o	chest
tonsill/o	tonsil
trache/o	windpipe; trachea
ur/o	urine or urea (waste material); urinary tract
vascul/o	blood vessel

III. Suffixes and Terminology

Suffixes are divided into two groups: those that describe **diagnoses** and those that describe **procedures.**

Diagnostic Suffixes

These suffixes describe disease conditions or their symptoms. Use the list of combining forms in the previous section to write the meaning of each term. You will find it helpful to check the meanings of the terms with the *Glossary of Medical Terms,* p. 313.

Noun Suffix	Meaning	Terminology	Meaning
-algia	condition of pain, pain	arthr<u>algia</u> _____	
		ot<u>algia</u> _____	
		my<u>algia</u> _____	
		neur<u>algia</u> _____	
-emia	blood condition	leuk<u>emia</u> _____	
		Increase in numbers of leukocytes; cells are malignant (cancerous).	
		septic<u>emia</u> _____	
		is<u>chemia</u> _____	
		Figure 3-1 illustrates ischemia of heart muscle caused by blockage of a coronary (heart) artery.	
		ur<u>emia</u> _____	
		Uremia occurs when the kidneys fail to function and urea (waste material) accumulates in the blood.	

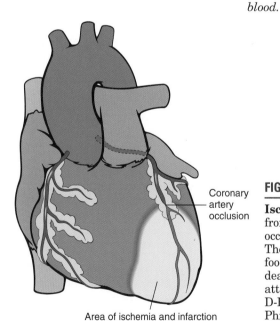

Coronary artery occlusion

Area of ischemia and infarction

FIGURE 3–1

Ischemia of heart muscle. Blood is held back from an area of the heart muscle by an occlusion (blockage) of a coronary (heart) artery. The muscle then loses its supply of oxygen and food and, if the condition persists, dies. The death of the heart muscle is known as a heart attack (myocardial infarction). (From Chabner D-E: _The Language of Medicine,_ ed 7, Philadelphia, 2004, WB Saunders.)

-ia   condition, disease   pneumonia _____

The lung is inflamed, and fluid or material collects in the air sacs of the lung.

-itis   inflammation   bronchitis _____

See Figure 3-2.

esophagitis _____

laryngitis _____

meningitis _____

The meninges are membranes that surround and protect the brain and spinal cord. See Figure 3-3.

cystitis _____

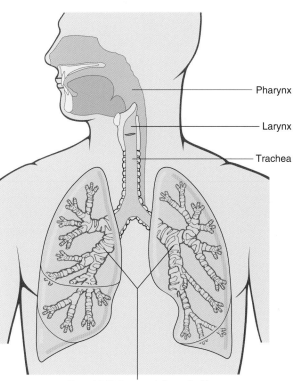

Pharynx

Larynx

Trachea

Bronchial tubes are inflamed with
hypersecretion of mucus

FIGURE 3–2

Bronchitis.

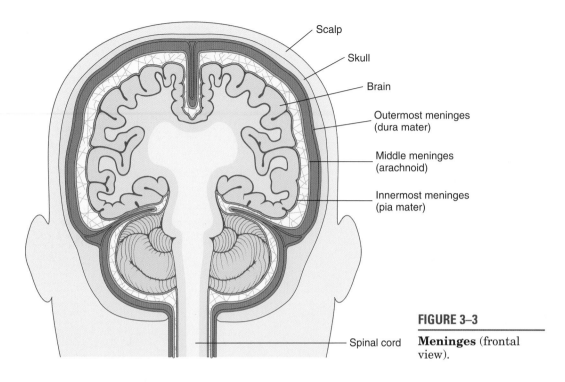

FIGURE 3–3

Meninges (frontal view).

phlebitis _____

colitis _____

Table 3-1 lists other common inflammatory conditions with their meanings.

-megaly	enlargement	cardiomegaly _____
		hepatomegaly _____
-oma	tumor, mass	adenoma _____

This is a benign (noncancerous) tumor.

adenocarcinoma _____

Carcinomas are malignant (cancerous) tumors of epithelial (skin or lining) tissue in the body. Glands and the linings of internal organs are composed of epithelial tissue.

myoma _____

This is a benign tumor.

TABLE 3–1	INFLAMMATIONS
appendicitis	Inflammation of the appendix (hangs from the colon in the lower right abdomen)
bursitis	Inflammation of a small sac of fluid (bursa) near a joint
cellulitis	Inflammation of soft tissue under the skin
dermatitis	Inflammation of the skin
endocarditis	Inflammation of the inner lining of the heart (endocardium)
epiglottitis	Inflammation of the epiglottis (cartilage at the upper part of the windpipe)
gastritis	Inflammation of the stomach
hepatitis	Inflammation of the liver
myositis	Inflammation of muscle (MYOS/O- means muscle)
nephritis	Inflammation of the kidney
osteomyelitis	Inflammation of bone and bone marrow
otitis	Inflammation of the ear
pharyngitis	Inflammation of the throat
thrombophlebitis	Inflammation of a vein with formation of clots

myosarc<u>oma</u> _____

Sarcomas are cancerous tumors of connective (flesh) tissue. Muscle, bone, cartilage, fibrous tissue, and fat are examples of connective tissues. See Table 3-2.

myel<u>oma</u> _____

MYEL/O- *means bone marrow in this term. Also called* **multiple myeloma,** *this is a malignant tumor of cells (called plasma cells) in the bone marrow. See Table 3-3 for names of other malignant tumors that do not contain the combining forms* CARCIN/O- *and* SARC/O-.

hemat<u>oma</u> _____

This is not a tumor but a collection of fluid (blood).

-osis   condition, abnormal condition   nephr<u>osis</u> _____

TABLE 3–2	SARCOMAS
chondrosarcoma	Cancer of cartilage tissue (CHONDR/O- means cartilage)
fibrosarcoma	Cancer of fibrous tissue (FIBR/O- means fibrous tissue)
leiomyosarcoma	Cancer of visceral (attached to internal organs) muscle (LEIOMY/O- means visceral muscle)
liposarcoma	Cancer of fatty tissue (LIP/O- means fat)
osteogenic sarcoma	Cancer of bone
rhabdomyosarcoma	Cancer of skeletal (attached to bones) muscle (RHABDOMY/O- means skeletal muscle)

3

TABLE 3–3	MALIGNANT TUMORS WHOSE NAMES DO NOT CONTAIN THE COMBINING FORMS CARCIN/O- AND SARC/O-
hepatoma	Malignant tumor of the liver *(hepatocellular carcinoma)*
lymphoma	Malignant tumor of lymph nodes (previously called *lymphosarcoma*)
melanoma	Malignant tumor of pigmented (MELAN/O- means black) cells in the skin
mesothelioma	Malignant tumor of pleural cells (membrane surrounding the lungs)
multiple myeloma	Malignant tumor of bone marrow cells
thymoma	Malignant tumor of the thymus gland (located in the mediastinum)

necrosis _____

erythrocytosis _____

When -OSIS is used with blood cell words, it means a slight increase in numbers of cells.

leukocytosis _____

This condition occurs as a normal response to infection.

-pathy   disease condition

encephalopathy _____

Pronunciation is en-sef-ah-**LOP**-ah-the.

cardiomyopathy _____

Pronunciation is kar-de-o-mi-**OP**-ah-the.

nephropathy _____

Pronunciation is neh-**FROP**-ah-the. *Table 3-4 lists other disease conditions.*

-rrhea   flow, discharge

rhinorrhea _____

menorrhea _____

Normal menstrual flow.

TABLE 3–4	DISEASE CONDITIONS (-PATHIES)
adrenopathy	Disease condition of the adrenal glands
hepatopathy	Disease condition of the liver
lymphadenopathy	Disease condition of the lymph nodes (previously called *glands*)
myopathy	Disease condition of muscles
neuropathy	Disease condition of nerves
osteopathy	Disease condition of bones
retinopathy	Disease condition of the retina of the eye

-rrhage or	bursting forth of blood	hemorrhage _____
-rrhagia		menorrhagia _____

Excessive bleeding during menstruation.

-sclerosis	hardening	arteriosclerosis _____

Atherosclerosis *is the most common type of arteriosclerosis. A fatty plaque (atheroma) collects on the lining of arteries. See Figure 3-4.*

-uria	condition of urine	hematuria _____

Bleeding into the urinary tract can cause this condition.

All the following **adjective suffixes** mean pertaining to and *describe* a part of the body, process, or condition.

-al or **-eal**	pertaining to	peritoneal _____
		inguinal _____

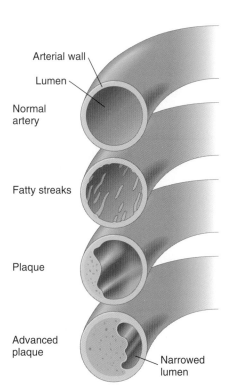

FIGURE 3–4

Atherosclerosis (type of arteriosclerosis). A fatty (cholesterol) material collects in an artery, narrowing it and eventually blocking the flow of blood.

renal _____

esophageal _____

myocardial _____

*A heart attack is also called a **myocardial infarction** (MI). An infarction is an area of dead tissue caused by ischemia (when blood supply is held back from a part of the body).*

-ar   pertaining to   vascular _____

*A **cerebrovascular accident (CVA)** is a stroke.*

-ary   pertaining to   axillary _____

mammary _____

pulmonary _____

-ic   pertaining to   chronic _____

*Chronic conditions occur over a long period of time, as opposed to **acute** conditions, which are sharp, sudden, and brief.*

pelvic _____

Procedural Suffixes

The following suffixes describe *procedures* used in patient care.

Suffix	Meaning	Terminology	Meaning
-centesis	surgical puncture to remove fluid	thoracentesis _____	
		The term is a shortened form of thoracocentesis. See Figure 3-5.	
		amniocentesis _____	
		See Figure 3-6.	
		arthrocentesis _____	
-ectomy	removal, resection, excision	tonsillectomy _____	
		Tonsils and adenoids are lymph tissue in the pharynx (throat). Lymph is composed of white blood cells that fight infection. See Figure 3-7.	

FIGURE 3–5

Technique of thoracentesis. A, The patient is sitting in the correct position for the procedure. **B,** The needle is advanced, and the fluid (pleural effusion) is drained.

FIGURE 3–6

Amniocentesis.

3

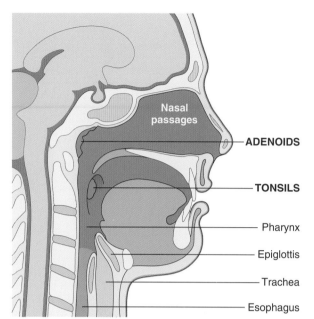

FIGURE 3–7

Tonsils and adenoids. A tonsillectomy and adenoidectomy (T&A) is removal of the tonsils and adenoids.

hysterectomy _____

*In a **total hysterectomy,** the whole uterus, including the cervix, is removed. If only a portion of the uterus is removed, the procedure is a* partial *or **subtotal hysterectomy.** See Figure 3-8.*

oophorectomy _____

salpingectomy _____

cholecystectomy _____
See Figure 3-9.

mastectomy _____
Table 3-5 lists additional resection procedures.

-gram   record   myelogram _____

MYEL/O- means spinal cord in this term. A contrast material is injected into the membranes around the spinal cord (by lumbar puncture), and then x-ray pictures are taken of the spinal cord. This procedure is performed less frequently now that MRI is available.

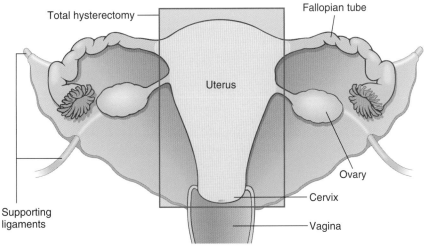

FIGURE 3–8

Total hysterectomy. In a total abdominal hysterectomy (TAH), the uterus is removed through the abdomen. A TAH-BSO is a total abdominal hysterectomy with bilateral salpingectomy and oophorectomy.

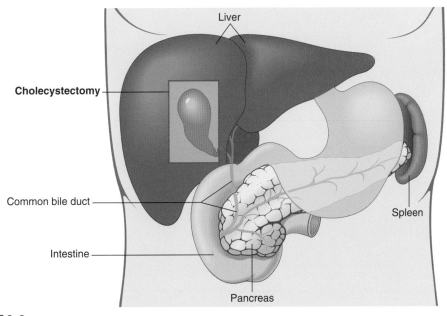

FIGURE 3–9

Cholecystectomy. The liver is lifted up to show the gallbladder underneath. The pancreas is a long, thin gland located behind and to the left of the stomach, toward the spleen. The common bile duct carries bile from the liver and gallbladder to the intestine.

TABLE 3–5	RESECTIONS
adenectomy	Excision of a gland
adenoidectomy	Excision of the adenoids
appendectomy	Excision of the appendix
colectomy	Excision of the colon
gastrectomy	Excision of the stomach
laminectomy	Excision of a piece of backbone (lamina) to relieve pressure on nerves from a (herniating) disk
myomectomy	Excision of a muscle tumor (commonly a fibroid of the uterus)
pneumonectomy	Excision of lung tissue; total pneumonectomy (an entire lung), or lobectomy (a single lobe)
splenectomy	Excision of the spleen

mammogram _____

See Figure 3-10.

-graphy　　　process of recording　　　electroencephalography _____

mammography _____

See Figure 3-11.

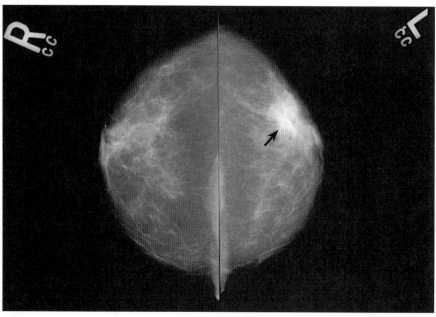

FIGURE 3–10

Mammograms of a 63-year-old woman. The right breast is normal, and the left breast contains a breast cancer *(arrow)*. (From Ballinger PW, Frank ED: *Merrill's Atlas of Radiographic Positions and Radiologic Procedures,* ed 10, vol 2, St Louis, 2003, Mosby.)

FIGURE 3–11

Mammography. The breast is compressed, and x-ray images (top to bottom and lateral) are taken. (From Ballinger PW and Frank ED: Merrill's Atlas of Radiographic Positions and Radiologic Procedures, Volume Two, 10th ed. St. Louis, Mosby, 2003, p. 510.)

angiography _____

Contrast material (such as iodine) is injected in an artery or vein and x-ray images are taken.

-lysis   separation,   dialysis _____
              breakdown,
              destruction   **Hemodialysis** *is the removal of blood and its passage through (DIA- means through or complete) a kidney machine to filter out waste materials, such as* urea. *Another form of dialysis is **peritoneal dialysis**. A special fluid is put into the peritoneum through a tube in the abdomen. The wastes seep into the fluid from the blood during a period of time. The fluid and wastes are then drained from the peritoneum. See Figure 3-12.*

FIGURE 3–12

Peritoneal dialysis. This procedure (or the alternative method of hemodialysis) is necessary when the kidneys are not functioning to remove waste materials (such as urea) from the blood. Without dialysis or kidney transplantation, uremia can result. (From Chabner D-E: *The Language of Medicine,* ed 7, Philadelphia, 2004, WB Saunders.)

-plasty	surgical repair, or surgical correction	mammo<u>plasty</u> _____
		rhino<u>plasty</u> _____
		angio<u>plasty</u> _____

*Balloon angioplasty is performed on the coronary arteries that surround the heart. A wire with a collapsed balloon is placed in a clogged artery. Opening of the balloon widens the vessel, allowing more blood to flow through. A **stent** (mesh rodlike device) is placed in the artery to hold it open. See Figure 3-13.*

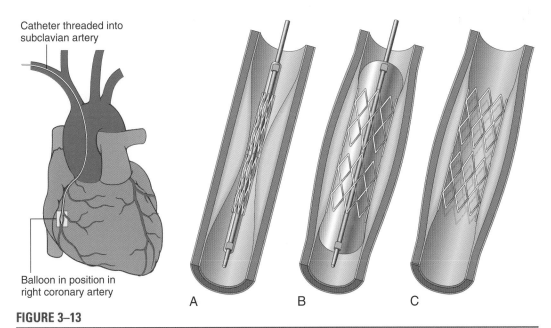

Catheter threaded into
subclavian artery

Balloon in position in
right coronary artery

A   B   C

FIGURE 3–13

Angioplasty and placement of an intracoronary artery stent. A, The stent is positioned at
the site of the lesion. **B,** The balloon is inflated, expanding the stent. **C,** The balloon is then
deflated and removed, and the implanted stent is left in place. Coronary artery stents are
stainless-steel scaffolding devices that help hold arteries open.

-scopy	process of visual examination	bronchoscopy _____
		laparoscopy _____
		laryngoscopy _____ _See Figure 3-14._
-stomy	opening	colostomy _____ _A -STOMY procedure is the creation of a permanent or semipermanent opening (stoma) from an organ to the outside of the body. See Figure 3-15. When two tubelike structures are surgically connected **within** the body, the new connection is an **anastomosis**. A **colocolostomy** is an anastomosis, a new connection between two previously unconnected portions of the colon._ tracheostomy _____ _See Figure 3-16, p. 95._

Larynx

FIGURE 3–14

Laryngoscopy.

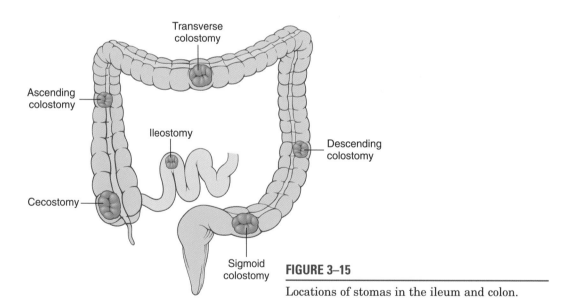

Transverse colostomy

Ascending colostomy

Ileostomy

Descending colostomy

Cecostomy

Sigmoid colostomy

FIGURE 3–15

Locations of stomas in the ileum and colon.

A   B

FIGURE 3–16

A, Tracheostomy with tube in place. **B, Healed tracheostomy incision** after laryngectomy.
(**B,** From Black JM, Matassarin-Jacobs E: *Medical-Surgical Nursing: Clinical Management for
Continuity of Care,* ed 5, Philadelphia, 1997, WB Saunders.)

-therapy	treatment	radio<u>therapy</u> _____
		chemo<u>therapy</u> _____
		cryo<u>therapy</u> _____

*Skin lesions, such as warts, are removed with
cryotherapy. Liquid nitrogen or carbon dioxide snow
is applied and blistering followed by necrosis results.*

| **-tomy** | incision, to cut into | cranio<u>tomy</u> _____ |

*-TOMY indicates a temporary incision, as opposed to
-STOMY, which is a permanent or semipermanent
opening.*

lapar<u>otomy</u> _____

phleb<u>otomy</u> _____
See Figure 3-17.

FIGURE 3–17

Phlebotomy. After entering a vein with a needle through the skin, the plunger of the syringe is pulled slowly to withdraw blood. (From Bonewit-West K: *Clinical Procedures for Medical Assistants,* ed 6, Philadelphia, 2004, WB Saunders.)

IV. Exercises and Answers

Complete these exercises and check your answers. An important part of your success in learning medical terminology is checking your answers carefully with the answer key beginning on p. 103.

A. Give meanings for the following suffixes:

1. -megaly _____

2. -pathy _____

3. -rrhea _____

4. -rrhagia _____

5. -osis _____

6. -ia _____

B. Give suffixes for the following English meanings:

1. inflammation _____

2. condition of pain _____

3. blood condition _____

4. tumor, mass _____

5. hardening _____

6. condition of urine _____

3

C. Match the following medical terms with their meanings below. Write each term next to its meaning.

adenocarcinoma	hepatomegaly	myeloma
cardiomyopathy	ischemia	otalgia
esophagitis	leukocytosis	pneumonia
hematoma		

1. Enlargement of the liver _____

2. Pain in the ear _____

3. Holding back blood from an organ (depriving it of blood supply) _____

4. Abnormal condition of white blood cells (slight increase in normal cells to fight

   infection) _____

5. Abnormal condition of the lung (inflammation and accumulation of material often

   caused by bacterial infection) _____

6. Tumor (malignant) of bone marrow _____

7. Inflammation of the tube leading from the throat to the stomach _____

8. Disease of heart muscle _____

9. Collection or mass of blood _____

10. Tumor (cancerous) of glandular tissue _____

D. Underline the suffix meaning <u>pertaining to</u> in the following terms and give the area or part of the body referred to:

1. esophageal _____

2. inguinal _____

3. renal _____

4. vascular _____

5. pelvic _____

6. pulmonary _____

7. axillary _____

8. peritoneal _____

9. mammary _____

10. myocardial _____

E. Give meanings for the following suffixes related to procedures:

1. -ectomy _____

2. -gram _____

3. -centesis _____

4. -graphy _____

5. -plasty _____

6. -lysis _____

7. -stomy _____

8. -scopy _____

9. -tomy _____

10. -therapy _____

F. Select from the following terms to complete the sentences below:

angiography   colocolostomy   mammogram
angioplasty   colostomy   oophorectomy
bronchoscopy   hysterectomy   phlebotomy
chemotherapy   laryngoscopy   thoracentesis

1. Surgical repair of a blood vessel using a catheter (tube), balloon, and stent is

   _____.

2. Treatment using chemicals to destroy malignant cells is _____.

3. X-ray record of the breast is a(an) _____.

4. Surgical puncture to remove fluid from the chest is _____.

5. A new opening of the large intestine to the outside of the body is a(an)

   _____.

6. A new internal connection (anastomosis) between two parts of the large bowel

   (intestine) is a(an) _____.

7. Removal of the uterus is a(an) _____.

8. Process of recording x-ray images of blood vessels after injecting contrast is

   _____.

9. Visual examination of the voice box is _____.

10. Incision of a vein to withdraw blood is _____.

G. Write the medical term for the following:

1. Bursting forth of blood _____

2. Hardening of fatty plaque (in the lining of the arteries) _____

3. Pertaining to time (occurring over a long period of time) _____

4. X-ray record of the spinal cord _____

5. Sharp, sudden, brief _____

6. Treatment using cold temperatures _____

7. Record of electricity in the brain _____

8. Surgical puncture to remove fluid from the membrane surrounding the fetus

_____

9. Muscle pain _____

10. Malignant tumor of bone marrow _____

11. Enlargement of the heart _____

12. Abnormal condition of the death of cells _____

13. Disease condition of the kidney _____

14. Incision of the skull _____

H. What part of the body is inflamed?

1. neuritis _____

2. arthritis _____

3. salpingitis _____

4. otitis _____

5. hepatitis _____

6. nephritis _____

7. esophagitis _____

8. laryngitis _____

9. encephalitis _____

10. osteitis _____

11. meningitis _____

12. bronchitis _____

13. rhinitis _____

14. peritonitis _____

15. vasculitis _____

16. mastitis _____

17. tonsillitis _____

18. colitis _____

19. pharyngitis _____

20. tracheitis _____

21. phlebitis _____

I. Provide the terms for the following procedures:

1. Excision of the gallbladder _____

2. Excision of the appendix _____

3. Excision of a breast _____

4. Excision of the uterus _____

5. Excision of an ovary _____

6. Excision of the voice box _____

7. Excision of a kidney _____

8. Excision of a gland _____

9. Excision of the large intestine _____

10. Excision of a fallopian tube _____

11. Excision of tonsils _____

12. Incision of the skull _____

13. Incision of the abdomen _____

14. Incision of the chest _____

15. Opening of the windpipe to the outside of the body _____

16. Opening of the colon to the outside of the body _____

17. Surgical puncture to remove fluid from the chest _____

18. Surgical puncture to remove fluid from a joint _____

19. Incision of a vein _____

20. Visual examination of the voice box _____

J. Supply the correct medical term for the following:

1. A stroke is a cerebro _____ _____ (two words).

2. A heart attack is a myo _____ _____ (two words).

3. Use of a machine that filters wastes from the blood is hemo _____.

4. Injection of fluid into the abdominal cavity and then withdrawal of that fluid

   (containing waste material) is peri _____ _____ (two words).

5. A noncancerous tumor of muscle is a my _____.

6. A cancerous tumor of muscle is a myo _____.

7. High levels of wastes (urea) in the blood is ur _____.

8. Blood in the urine is hemat _____.

9. High numbers of malignant (cancerous) white blood cells is leuk _____.

10. Slightly elevated numbers of white blood cells due to an infection in the body is

    leuko _____.

11. Normal discharge of blood during menstruation is men _____.

12. Excessive bleeding during menstruation is men _____.

13. Hardening of arteries is called arterio _____.

14. Use of high-energy rays to treat cancerous tumors is radio _____.

K. Circle the term that best completes the meaning of the sentences in the following medical vignettes:

1. After routine breast self-examination, Nora felt a small lump in her breast. She consulted her doctor who scheduled a diagnostic **(mammoplasty, mastectomy, mammogram).** The examination showed a stellate (star-shaped) mass and a **(biopsy, necropsy, laparoscopy)** revealed an infiltrating ductal carcinoma. Nora decided to have her breast removed **(hysterectomy, mastectomy, salpingectomy)**, although her physician gave her the option of having lumpectomy followed by **(cryotherapy, thoracotomy, radiotherapy).**

2. In addition to her surgery, Nora had a sentinel node biopsy of a (an) **(inguinal, thoracic, axillary)** lymph node to determine whether the cancer had spread. Injection of contrast revealed the primary (sentinel) lymph node, which was removed and microscopically examined.

3

3. Sylvia had irregular bleeding in between her periods. She was 50 years old and beginning menopause. On pelvic exam, Dr. Hawk felt a large, lobulated uterus. Biopsy revealed a large fibroid, which is a benign (noncancerous) tumor of muscle tissue **(myeloma, myoma, hematoma)**. The doctor suggested a total abdominal **(gastrectomy, hysterectomy, cholecystectomy)**.

4. Victoria had never been comfortable with the bump on her nose. She saw a plastic surgeon, who performed **(mammoplasty, rhinoplasty, angioplasty)**.

5. Sam was experiencing cramps, diarrhea, and a low-grade fever. He was diagnosed with ulcerative **(colitis, meningitis, laryngitis)** and had several bouts of **(uremia, menorrhagia, septicemia)** caused by inflammation and rupture of the bowel wall.

6. Bill felt chest pain every time he climbed a flight of stairs. He went to his doctor, who did a coronary **(myelogram, angiogram, dialysis)** that revealed **(adenocarcinoma, nephrosis, atherosclerosis)** in one of his coronary arteries. The doctor recommended **(angioplasty, thoracentesis, amniocentesis)**. This would prevent further **(myosarcoma, ischemia, leukocytosis)** and help Bill avoid a **(peritoneal, vascular, myocardial)** infarction, or heart attack, in the future.

Answers to Exercises

A

1. enlargement
2. disease condition
3. flow, discharge
4. bursting forth of blood
5. condition, abnormal condition
6. condition, disease

B

1. -itis   2. -algia   3. -emia   4. -oma   5. -sclerosis   6. -uria

C

1. hepatomegaly
2. otalgia
3. ischemia
4. leukocytosis
5. pneumonia
6. myeloma (also called multiple myeloma)
7. esophagitis
8. cardiomyopathy
9. hematoma
10. adenocarcinoma

D

1. esophag**eal**—esophagus (tube leading from the throat to the stomach)
2. inguin**al**—groin (area where the thigh meets the trunk of the body)
3. ren**al**—kidney
4. vascul**ar**—blood vessels
5. pelv**ic**—hip area
6. pulmon**ary**—lungs
7. axill**ary**—arm pit (underarm area)
8. periton**eal**—peritoneum (membrane surrounding the abdominal cavity)
9. mamm**ary**—breast
10. myocardi**al**—heart muscle

E

1. removal, excision, resection
2. record
3. surgical puncture to remove fluid
4. process of recording
5. surgical repair
6. separation; breakdown
7. new opening
8. process of visual examination
9. cut into, incision, section
10. treatment

F

1. angioplasty
2. chemotherapy
3. mammogram
4. thoracentesis
5. colostomy
6. colocolostomy
7. hysterectomy
8. angiography
9. laryngoscopy
10. phlebotomy

G

1. hemorrhage
2. atherosclerosis
3. chronic
4. myelogram
5. acute
6. cryotherapy
7. electroencephalogram
8. amniocentesis
9. myalgia
10. myeloma or multiple myeloma
11. cardiomegaly
12. necrosis
13. nephropathy
14. craniotomy

H

1. nerve
2. joint
3. fallopian tubes
4. ear
5. liver
6. kidney
7. esophagus
8. larynx (voice box)
9. brain
10. bone
11. meninges (membranes surrounding the brain and spinal cord)
12. bronchial tubes
13. nose
14. peritoneum
15. blood vessels
16. breast
17. tonsils
18. colon (large intestine)
19. throat (pharynx)
20. trachea (windpipe)
21. veins

3

I

1. cholecystectomy
2. appendectomy
3. mastectomy
4. hysterectomy
5. oophorectomy
6. laryngectomy
7. nephrectomy
8. adenectomy
9. colectomy
10. salpingectomy
11. tonsillectomy
12. craniotomy
13. laparotomy
14. thoracotomy
15. tracheostomy
16. colostomy
17. thoracentesis
18. arthrocentesis
19. phlebotomy
20. laryngoscopy

J

1. cerebro**vascular accident**—clot or hemorrhage in an artery of the brain leads to decreased blood flow (ischemia) to brain tissue and necrosis (death of brain cells).
2. myo**cardial infarction**—ischemia to heart muscle leads to infarction (death or necrosis of heart muscle cells).
3. hemo**dialysis**—complete separation of waste material from the blood using a machine that receives the patient's blood and after filtration sends the blood back into the patient's body.
4. peri**toneal dialysis**—fluid is introduced into the abdominal cavity and then removed after wastes have passed into the fluid from the peritoneal blood vessels.
5. my**oma**—benign muscle tumors occurring in the uterus are fibroids.
6. myo**sarcoma**—malignant tumors of connective or flesh tissue are sarcomas.
7. ur**emia**—this indicates failure of the kidneys to eliminate nitrogen-containing wastes, such as urea, creatinine, and uric acid from the bloodstream.
8. hemat**uria**—this indicates bleeding in the urinary tract.
9. leuk**emia**—immature, cancerous white blood cells are produced in excess from the bone marrow or lymph nodes.
10. leuko**cytosis**—normal, mature white blood cells are produced to fight infection.
11. men**orrhea**—lining of the uterus breaks down due to changes in hormone levels.
12. men**orrhagia**—long or heavy menstrual periods; often caused by benign muscle tumors or fibroids in the uterus.
13. arterio**sclerosis**—the most common type is atherosclerosis or collection of fatty plaques in arteries.
14. radio**therapy**—using high energy x-rays, gamma rays, or protons to destroy cancerous cells.

K

1. mammogram, biopsy, mastectomy, radiotherapy
2. axillary
3. myoma, hysterectomy
4. rhinoplasty
5. colitis, septicemia
6. angiogram, atherosclerosis, angioplasty, ischemia, myocardial

V. Review

Write the meanings for the following word parts. Remember to check your answers with the Answers to Review on p. 108.

Suffixes

Suffix	Meaning	Suffix	Meaning
1. -al		15. -megaly	
2. -algia		16. -oma	
3. -ar		17. -osis	
4. -ary		18. -pathy	
5. -centesis		19. -plasty	
6. -eal		20. -rrhage	
7. -ectomy		21. -rrhagia	
8. -emia		22. -rrhea	
9. -gram		23. -sclerosis	
10. -graphy		24. -scopy	
11. -ia		25. -stomy	
12. -ic		26. -therapy	
13. -itis		27. -tomy	
14. -lysis		28. -uria	

Combining Forms

Combining Form	Meaning	Combining Form	Meaning
1. aden/o		2. amni/o	

3. angi/o _____

4. arteri/o _____

5. arthr/o _____

6. ather/o _____

7. axill/o _____

8. bronch/o _____

9. carcin/o _____

10. cardi/o _____

11. chem/o _____

12. cholecyst/o _____

13. chron/o _____

14. col/o _____

15. crani/o _____

16. cry/o _____

17. cyst/o _____

18. encephal/o _____

19. erythr/o _____

20. esophag/o _____

21. hemat/o _____

22. hepat/o _____

23. hyster/o _____

24. inguin/o _____

25. isch/o _____

26. lapar/o _____

27. laryng/o _____

28. leuk/o _____

29. mamm/o _____

30. mast/o _____

31. men/o _____

32. mening/o _____

33. my/o _____

34. myel/o _____

35. necr/o _____

36. nephr/o _____

37. neur/o _____

38. oophor/o _____

39. oste/o _____

40. ot/o _____

41. pelv/o _____

42. peritone/o _____

43. phleb/o _____

44. pneumon/o _____

45. pulmon/o _____

46. radi/o _____

47. ren/o _____

48. rhin/o _____

3

49. salping/o _____

50. sarc/o _____

51. septic/o _____

52. thorac/o _____

53. tonsill/o _____

54. trache/o _____

55. ur/o _____

56. vascul/o _____

Answers to Review

Suffixes

1. pertaining to
2. condition of pain, pain
3. pertaining to
4. pertaining to
5. surgical puncture to remove fluid
6. pertaining to
7. removal, resection, excision
8. blood condition
9. record
10. process of recording
11. condition
12. pertaining to
13. inflammation
14. separation, breakdown, destruction
15. enlargement
16. tumor, mass
17. abnormal condition
18. disease condition
19. surgical repair
20. bursting forth of blood
21. bursting forth of blood
22. flow, discharge
23. hardening
24. visual examination
25. opening
26. treatment
27. incision; to cut into
28. urine condition

Combining Forms

1. gland
2. amnion
3. vessel
4. artery
5. joint
6. plaque, collection of fatty material
7. armpit
8. bronchial tubes
9. cancerous
10. heart
11. drug, chemical
12. gallbladder
13. time
14. colon (large intestine)
15. skull
16. cold
17. urinary bladder
18. brain
19. red
20. esophagus
21. blood
22. liver
23. uterus
24. groin
25. to hold back
26. abdomen
27. larynx (voice box)
28. white
29. breast
30. breast
31. menstruation
32. meninges
33. muscle
34. spinal cord or bone marrow
35. death
36. kidney
37. nerve
38. ovary
39. bone
40. ear
41. hip area
42. peritoneum
43. vein
44. lung
45. lung
46. x-rays
47. kidney
48. nose
49. fallopian tube
50. flesh
51. pertaining to infection
52. chest
53. tonsil
54. trachea (windpipe)
55. urine, urinary tract
56. blood vessel

VI. Pronunciation of Terms

The terms that you have learned in this chapter are presented here with their pronunciations. The capitalized letters in boldface are the accented syllable. Pronounce each word out loud, then write the meaning in the space provided. Meanings of all terms can be checked with the *Glossary of Medical Terms*, p. 313.

Term	Pronunciation	Meaning
acute	ah-**KUT**	
adenocarcinoma	ah-deh-no-kar-sih-**NO**-mah	
adenoma	ah-deh-**NO**-mah	
amniocentesis	am-ne-o-sen-**TE**-sis	
anastomosis	ah-nah-sto-**MO**-sis	
angiography	an-je-**OG**-rah-fe	
angioplasty	**AN**-je-o-plas-te	
arteriosclerosis	ar-ter-e-o-skle-**RO**-sis	
arthralgia	ar-**THRAL**-je-ah	
arthropathy	ar-**THROP**-ah-the	
atherosclerosis	ah-theh-ro-skle-**RO**-sis	
axillary	**AKS**-ih-lar-e	
bronchitis	brong-**KI**-tis	
bronchoscopy	brong-**KOS**-ko-pe	
carcinoma	kar-sih-**NO**-mah	
cardiomegaly	kar-de-o-**MEG**-ah-le	
cardiomyopathy	kar-de-o-mi-**OP**-ah-the	
chemotherapy	ke-mo-**THER**-ah-pe	

cholecystectomy	ko-le-sis-**TEK**-to-me _____
chronic	**KRON**-ik _____
colitis	ko-**LI**-tis _____
colostomy	ko-**LOS**-to-me _____
colocolostomy	ko-lo-ko-**LOS**-to-me _____
craniotomy	kra-ne-**OT**-o-me _____
cystitis	sis-**TI**-tis _____
dialysis	di-**AL**-ih-sis _____
electroencephalography	e-lek-tro-en-sef-ah-**LOG**-rah-fe _____
encephalopathy	en-sef-ah-**LOP**-ah-the _____
erythrocytosis	eh-rith-ro-si-**TO**-sis _____
esophageal	e-sof-ah-**JE**-al _____
esophagitis	e-sof-ah-**JI**-tis _____
hematoma	he-mah-**TO**-mah _____
hematuria	he-mah-**TUR**-e-ah _____
hemorrhage	**HEM**-or-ij _____
hysterectomy	his-teh-**REK**-to-me _____
infarction	in-**FARK**-shun _____
inguinal	**ING**-gwi-nal _____
ischemia	is-**KE**-me-ah _____
laparoscopy	lap-ah-**ROS**-ko-pe _____
laparotomy	lap-ah-**ROT**-o-me _____
laryngitis	lah-rin-**JI**-tis _____

laryngoscopy	lah-rin-**GOS**-ko-pe	_____
leukemia	lu-**KE**-me-ah	_____
leukocytosis	lu-ko-si-**TO**-sis	_____
mammogram	**MAM**-o-gram	_____
mammography	mam-**MOG**-rah-fe	_____
mammoplasty	**MAM**-o-plas-te	_____
mastectomy	mas-**TEK**-to-me	_____
meningitis	men-in-**JI**-tis	_____
menorrhagia	men-or-**RA**-jah	_____
menorrhea	men-o-**RE**-ah	_____
myalgia	mi-**AL**-jah	_____
myelogram	**MI**-eh-lo-gram	_____
myeloma	mi-eh-**LO**-mah	_____
myocardial	mi-o-**KAR**-de-al	_____
myoma	mi-**O**-mah	_____
myosarcoma	mi-o-sar-**KO**-mah	_____
necrosis	neh-**KRO**-sis	_____
nephrosis	neh-**FRO**-sis	_____
neuralgia	nu-**RAL**-jah	_____
oophorectomy	o-of-o-**REK**-to-me or oo-for-**REK**-to-me	_____
otalgia	o-**TAL**-jah	_____
pelvic	**PEL**-vik	_____
peritoneal	per-ih-to-**NE**-al	_____

3

3

phlebitis	fleh-**BI**-tis _____
phlebotomy	fleh-**BOT**-o-me _____
pneumonia	noo-**MO**-ne-ah _____
pulmonary	**PUL**-mo-ner-re _____
radiotherapy	ra-de-o-**THER**-ah-pe _____
renal	**RE**-nal _____
rhinoplasty	**RI**-no-plas-te _____
rhinorrhea	ri-no-**RE**-ah _____
salpingectomy	sal-ping-**JEK**-to-me _____
septicemia	sep-tih-**SE**-me-ah _____
thoracentesis	tho-rah-sen-**TE**-sis _____
tonsillectomy	ton-sih-**LEK**-to-me _____
tracheostomy	tra-ke-**OS**-to-me _____
uremia	u-**RE**-me-ah _____
vascular	**VAS**-ku-lar _____

VII. Practical Applications

Answers are found on p. 114.

A. Match the procedure in Column I with an abnormal condition it treats or diagnoses in Column II:

Column I Procedure		Column II Abnormal Condition or Diagnosis
1. angioplasty	_____	A. uterine adenocarcinoma
2. mammoplasty	_____	B. ligament tear of the patella (knee cap)

3. cholecystectomy _____   C. ovarian cyst

4. tonsillectomy   _____   D. blockage of the windpipe

5. dialysis   _____   E. renal failure

6. hysterectomy   _____   F. absence of a breast (postmastectomy)

7. thoracentesis   _____   G. pleural effusion (collection of fluid)

8. oophorectomy   _____   H. coronary atherosclerosis

9. tracheostomy   _____   I. gallbladder calculi (stones)

10. arthroscopy   _____   J. pharyngeal lymph node enlargement

B. Match the symptom or abnormal condition in Column I with an organ or tissue in Column II:

Column I Symptom or Abnormal Condition	Column II Organ or Tissue

1. colitis   _____   A. uterus

2. phlebitis   _____   B. ear

3. menorrhagia   _____   C. bone marrow

4. myocardial ischemia _____   D. coronary arteries

5. otalgia   _____   E. large bowel

6. uremia   _____   F. spinal cord or brain

7. meningitis   _____   G. vein

8. leukemia   _____   H. kidney

Answers to Practical Applications

A

1. H	3. I	5. E	7. G	9. D
2. F	4. J	6. A	8. C	10. B

B

1. E	3. A	5. B	7. F
2. G	4. D	6. H	8. C

VIII. Picture Show

Answer the questions that follow each image. Correct answers are found on p. 116.

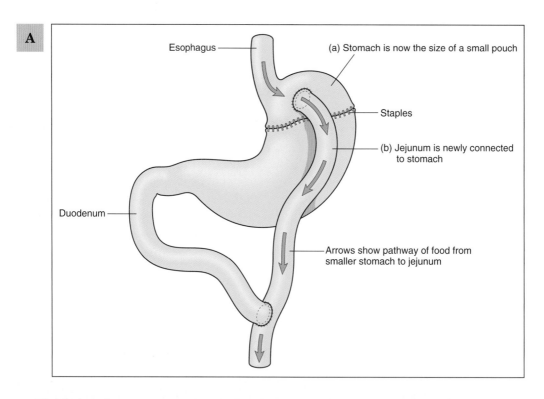

A

Esophagus

(a) Stomach is now the size of a small pouch

Staples

(b) Jejunum is newly connected to stomach

Duodenum

Arrows show pathway of food from smaller stomach to jejunum

1. The figure shows a surgical procedure to treat extreme obesity. First, the stomach (a) is stapled so that it is reduced to the size of a small pouch. Next, the jejunum (b), which is the second part of the small intestine, is brought up to connect with

the smaller stomach. This diverts food so that it has a shorter travel time through the intestine and less food is absorbed into the bloodstream. What is the name of this surgical procedure?

a. esophageal bypass

c. gastric bypass

b. total gastric resection

d. duodenal resection

2. The new connection, or anastomosis, between the stomach and the second part of the small intestine is a

a. gastrostomy

c. gastroduodenostomy

b. jejunostomy

d. gastrojejunostomy

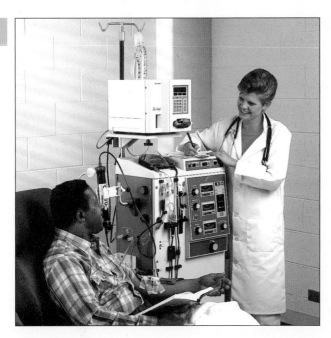

(From Lewis SM, Heitkemper MM, Dirksen SR: *Medical-Surgical Nursing: Assessment and Management of Clinical Problems,* ed 5, St Louis, 2000, Mosby.)

1. In the procedure above, blood leaves the patient's body to enter a machine that filters out impurities. The filtered blood then circulates back to the patient's body. This procedure is

a. pericardiocentesis

c. hemodialysis

b. peritoneal dialysis

d. amniocentesis

2. The procedure treats patients with failure of the

a. kidneys

c. liver

b. pancreas

d. all of the above

C

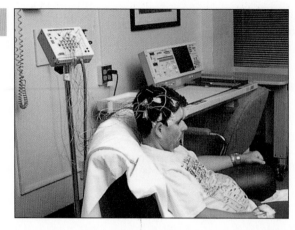

(From Chipps EM, Clanin NJ, Campbell VG: *Neurologic Disorders,* St Louis, 1992, Mosby.)

1. This procedure records brain wave activity. It is

    a. electrocardiography   c. electromyography
    b. electroencephalography   d. electrocraniography

2. It may be used to diagnose

    a. seizure disorders (epilepsy)   d. quadriplegia
    b. dyspnea   e. all of the above
    c. paraplegia

Answers to Picture Show

A

1. c   2. d

B

1. c   2. a

C

1. b   2. a

IX. Medical Scramble

Unscramble the letters to form a medical term from the clues. Use the letters in squares to complete the bonus term. Answers are upside down at the bottom of the page.

1. Suffix meaning enlargement

— ☐ __ __ __ __ __   G A Y M L E

2. Suffix meaning separation, breakdown

— ☐ __ __ __ __   S Y S I L

3. Holding back blood from an area of the body

__ __ __ __ __ ☐ __ __   H A S E I M I C

4. Ear pain

☐ __ __ __ __ __ __   T A I L O G A

5. Benign tumor of muscle

__ ☐ __ __ __   Y M O A M

6. Sharp, sudden, severe

☐ __ __ __ ☐   T U E C A

BONUS TERM: TUMOR OF BONE MARROW
(hint: it affects MULTIPLE areas of bone marrow tissue)

☐ ☐ ☐ ☐ ☐ ☐ ☐

4

Prefixes

Chapter Sections

Chapter Objectives

- To identify and define common prefixes used in medical terms
- To analyze, spell, and pronounce medical terms that contain prefixes

I. Introduction

This chapter reviews the prefixes you studied in Chapter 1 and introduces new prefixes. The list of Combining Forms and Suffixes that follows in Section II will help you understand the terminology in Section III. Complete all Exercises in Section IV and check your answers. The Review and the Pronunciation of Terms are opportunities to test your understanding of all the terminology in this chapter.

II. Combining Forms and Suffixes

Combining Form	Meaning
abdomin/o	abdomen
an/o	anus (opening of the digestive tract to the outside of the body)
bi/o	life
cardi/o	heart
carp/o	carpals (wrist bones)
cis/o	to cut
cost/o	ribs
crani/o	skull
cutane/o	skin
dur/o	dura mater (outermost meningeal membrane surrounding the brain and spinal cord)
gen/o	to produce, to begin
glyc/o	sugar
hemat/o	blood
later/o	side
men/o	menses (monthly discharge of blood from the lining of the uterus)
nat/i	birth
neur/o	nerve
norm/o	rule, order
oste/o	bone
peritone/o	peritoneum (membrane surrounding the organs in the abdomen)
plas/o	formation, growth, development
ren/o	kidney
scapul/o	scapula (shoulder blade)
son/o	sound
thyroid/o	thyroid gland
top/o	to put, place, position
troph/o	development, nourishment

urethr/o	urethra (tube leading from the bladder to the outside of the body)
uter/o	uterus
ven/o	vein
vertebr/o	vertebra (backbone)

Suffix	Meaning
-al	pertaining to
-ation	process, condition
-cision	process of cutting
-crine	secretion
-dipsia	thirst
-emia	blood condition
-gen	to produce
-graphy	process of recording
-ia	condition, process
-ic	pertaining to
-ine	pertaining to
-ism	condition, process
-lapse	to fall, slide
-lysis	loosening, breakdown, separation, destruction
-mission	to send
-mortem	death
-oma	tumor, mass
-ous	pertaining to
-partum	birth
-pathy	disease condition
-phagia	to eat, swallow
-phasia	to speak
-plasm	formation
-plegia	paralysis
-pnea	breathing
-rrhea	flow, discharge
-scopy	process of visual examination
-section	to cut
-stasis	to stand, place, stop, control
-tension	pressure
-thesis	to put, place (state of putting or placing)
-tic	pertaining to
-um	structure
-uria	urine condition
-y	process, condition

III. Prefixes and Terminology

Prefix	Meaning	Terminology	Meaning
a-, an-	no, not, without	apnea _____	
		aphasia _____	
			A stroke on the left side of the brain can produce this condition.
		atrophy _____	
			Disuse of a muscle can result in muscular atrophy. Muscles shrink as cells decrease in size.
		anemia _____	
			Anemia is a condition in which there is a lower-than-normal number of red blood cells or a decrease in hemoglobin in the cells. Table 4-1 lists different forms of anemia.
		amenorrhea _____	
ab-	away from	abnormal _____	

TABLE 4–1	ANEMIAS
aplastic anemia	Bone marrow fails to produce red blood cells (erythrocytes), white blood cells (leukocytes), and clotting cells (platelets).
hemolytic anemia	Red blood cells are destroyed (-LYTIC), and bone marrow cannot compensate for their loss. This condition can be hereditary or acquired (after infection or chemotherapy) or can occur when the immune system acts against normal red blood cells (autoimmune condition).
iron deficiency anemia	Low or absent iron levels lead to low hemoglobin concentration or deficiency of red blood cells.
pernicious anemia	The mucous membrane of the stomach fails to produce a factor (intrinsic factor) that is necessary for the absorption of vitamin B_{12} and the proper formation of red blood cells.
sickle cell anemia	Erythrocytes assume an abnormal crescent or sickle shape; it is caused by the inheritance of an abnormal type of hemoglobin. The sickle-shaped cells clump together, causing clots that block blood vessels.

FIGURE 4–1

Adrenal glands. These two endocrine glands are above each kidney. (Modified from Chabner D-E: *The Language of Medicine,* ed 7, Philadelphia, 2004, WB Saunders.)

ad-	toward, near	adrenal glands _____
		Adrenal glands are also called suprarenal (SUPRA-means above) glands. See Figure 4-1.
ana-	up, apart	analysis _____
		A urinalysis (urine + analysis) is a separation of urine to determine its contents.
ante-	before, forward	antepartum _____
anti-	against	antibody _____
		An antibody is a protein made by white blood cells; literally, a "body" working "against" foreign substances.
		antigen _____
		Antigens are foreign substances, such as bacteria and viruses. When antigens enter the body, they stimulate white blood cells to produce antibodies that act against the antigens.

4

4

antibiotic _____

Antibiotics differ from antibodies in that they are produced outside the body by microorganisms and primitive plants called molds. Examples of antibiotics are penicillin and erythromycin.

bi- two, both bilateral _____

brady- slow bradycardia _____

con- with, together congenital _____

A congenital anomaly is an irregularity (anomaly) present at birth. Examples are webbed fingers and toes and heart defects.

dia- through, complete diarrhea _____

dialysis _____

-LYSIS means separation here.

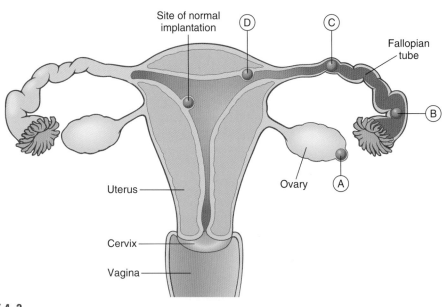

FIGURE 4–2

Ectopic pregnancy. A, B, C, and **D** are ectopic sites. The fallopian tube is the most common site for ectopic pregnancies (95%), but they can also occur on the ovary or on the surface of the peritoneum. Normal implantation takes place on the inner lining (endometrium) of the uterus.

dys-	bad, painful, difficult, abnormal	dyspnea _____
		dysphagia _____
		dysplasia _____
		dysmenorrhea _____
		dysuria _____
ec-	out, outside	ectopic pregnancy _____

Figure 4-2 shows possible sites of ectopic pregnancies. Figure 4-3 indicates uterine levels in a normal pregnancy.

endo-	within, in, inner	endoscopy _____

Table 4-2 lists examples of endoscopies.

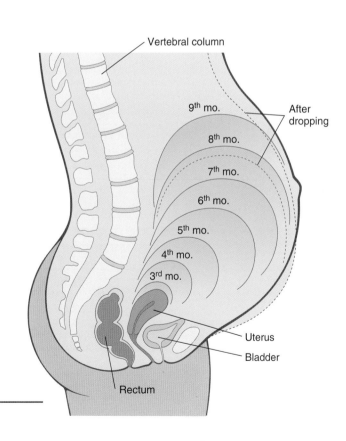

FIGURE 4–3

Uterine levels in pregnancy.

TABLE 4–2	ENDOSCOPIES
arthroscopy	Visual examination of a joint
bronchoscopy	Visual examination of the bronchial tubes
colonoscopy	Visual examination of the colon (large intestine)
cystoscopy	Visual examination of the urinary bladder
esophagoscopy	Visual examination of the esophagus
gastroscopy	Visual examination of the stomach
hysteroscopy	Visual examination of the uterus
laparoscopy	Visual examination of the abdomen
laryngoscopy	Visual examination of the larynx (voice box)
mediastinoscopy	Visual examination of the mediastinum
proctosigmoidoscopy	Visual examination of the rectum and sigmoid colon
sigmoidoscopy	Visual examination of the sigmoid colon (lower, S-shaped part of the large intestine)

endocrine glands _____

The adrenal glands are endocrine glands. Table 4-3 lists the major endocrine glands and the hormones they secrete.

epi-   above, upon   epidural hematoma _____

Figure 4-4 illustrates epidural and subdural hematomas.

epidermis _____

The three layers of the skin, from outermost to innermost, are the epidermis, dermis, and subcutaneous layer. Check Appendix I for a diagram of the skin.

TABLE 4–3	MAJOR ENDOCRINE GLANDS AND SELECTED HORMONES	
	Gland	**Hormones**
	adrenal glands	Adrenaline (epinephrine)
	ovaries	Estrogen
		Progesterone
	pancreas	Insulin
	parathyroid glands	Parathyroid hormone (PTH)
	pituitary gland	Adrenocorticotrophic hormone (ACTH)
		Follicle-stimulating hormone (FSH)
		Growth hormone (GH)
		Thyroid-stimulating hormone (TSH)
	testes	Testosterone
	thyroid gland	Thyroxine (T_4)

SUBDURAL HEMATOMA   Dura mater

Head injury

Skull

EPIDURAL
HEMATOMA

Brain

Brain tissue

4

FIGURE 4–4

Epidural and subdural hematomas. The dura mater is the outermost of the three meninges (membranes) around the brain and spinal cord.

ex-	out	excision _____
extra-	outside of	extrahepatic _____
hemi-	half	hemigastrectomy _____

hemiplegia _____
One side of the body is paralyzed; usually caused by a cerebrovascular accident or brain lesion, such as a tumor. The paralysis occurs on the side opposite the brain disorder.

hyper-	excessive, too much, above	hyperthyroidism _____

Figure 4-5 shows the position of the thyroid gland in the neck.

hypertrophy _____
*Cells increase in size, not in number. The opposite of hypertrophy is **atrophy** (cells shrink in size).*

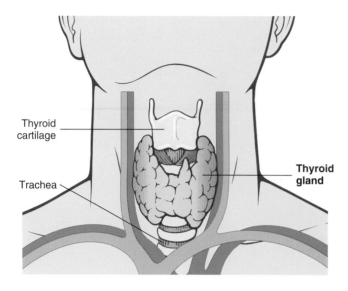

Thyroid cartilage

Trachea

Thyroid gland

FIGURE 4–5

Thyroid gland, located in the front of the trachea in the neck. The thyroid gland produces too much hormone in hyperthyroidism.

hypertension _____

Risk factors that contribute to high blood pressure are increasing age, smoking, obesity, heredity, and a stressful lifestyle.

hyperglycemia _____

Also known as diabetes mellitus. Insulin is either not secreted or improperly utilized so that sugar accumulates in the bloodstream and spills over into the urine (glycosuria).

hypo-   deficient, too little, below

hypoglycemia _____

Overproduction of insulin or an overdose (from outside the body—exogenously) of insulin can lead to hypoglycemia, as glucose is removed from the blood at an increased rate.

in-   in, into

incision _____

inter-   between

intervertebral _____

intra-   within

intrauterine _____

intravenous _____

mal-   bad

malignant _____

*-IGNANT comes from the Latin ignis, meaning "fire." A malignant tumor is a cancerous growth. A **benign** tumor (ben means "good") is a noncancerous growth.*

meta-   change, beyond

metastasis _____

This term literally means a "change of place" (-STASIS). It is the spread of a cancerous tumor from its original place to a secondary location in the body.

metacarpals _____

*The carpal bones are the wrist bones, and the metacarpals are the hand bones, which are **beyond** the wrist. See the x-ray image of the hand in Figure 4-6.*

neo-   new

neoplasm _____

neoplastic _____

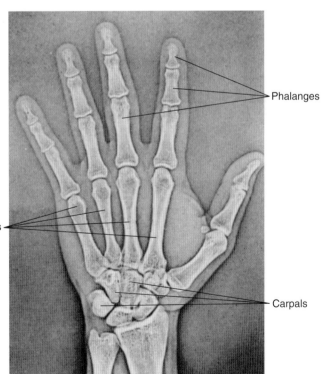

FIGURE 4–6

Metacarpals. This x-ray film of a hand shows metacarpals, carpals (wrist bones), and phalanges (finger bones).

A   B

FIGURE 4–7

Neonates in the neonatal intensive care unit (NICU). A, Benjamin Oliver Chabner, born May 22, 2001, at 32 weeks (8 weeks premature). **B,** Samuel August Thompson, born August 13, 2001, at 36 weeks. Gus needed an endotracheal tube through which he received surfactant, a substance necessary to inflate his lungs. Both children are healthy and a delight to their grandmother.

neonatal _____

Neonates who are born prematurely are often treated in the neonatal intensive care unit (NICU). See Figure 4-7.

para-   beside, near, along the side of

parathyroid glands _____

Figure 4-8 shows the position of the parathyroid glands on the back side of the thyroid gland. The parathyroid glands are endocrine glands that regulate the amount of calcium in bones and in the blood.

paralysis _____

This term came from the Greek paralyikos, *meaning "one whose side was loose or weak," as after a stroke. Now it means a loss of movement in any part of the body caused by a break in the connection between nerve and muscle.*

paraplegia _____

-PLEGIA *means paralysis, and this term originally meant paralysis of any limb or side of the body. Since the nineteenth century, however, it has indicated paralysis of the lower half of the body.*

4

FIGURE 4–8

Parathyroid glands. These are four endocrine glands on the posterior (back side) of the thyroid gland.

peri-	surrounding	periosteum _____
		perianal _____
poly-	many, much	polyuria _____
		polyneuropathy _____
		polydipsia _____
		Symptoms of diabetes mellitus are polyuria and polydipsia.
post-	after, behind	postpartum _____
		postmortem _____
pre-	before	precancerous _____
		prenatal _____
pro-	before, forward	prolapse _____
		-LAPSE means to slide. Figure 4-9 shows both the normal position of the uterus and its position when prolapsed.

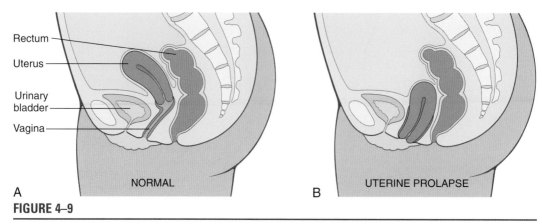

Rectum

Uterus

Urinary bladder

Vagina

A   NORMAL

B   UTERINE PROLAPSE

FIGURE 4–9

Prolapsed uterus. Prolapsed uterus is shown in **B.** Normally, the uterus is tilted forward above the urinary bladder **(A).**

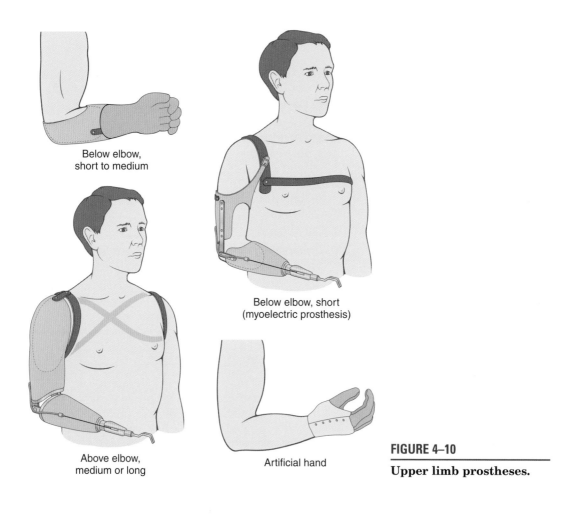

Below elbow, short to medium

Below elbow, short (myoelectric prosthesis)

Above elbow, medium or long

Artificial hand

FIGURE 4–10

Upper limb prostheses.

pros-	before, forward	prosthesis _____
		An artificial limb is a prosthesis (literally meaning "to put before or forward"). Figure 4-10 illustrates several types of prostheses. Figure 4-11 shows a total hip replacement and a total knee joint replacement.
quadri-	four	quadriplegia _____
		Paralysis of all four limbs.
re-	back, behind	relapse _____
		Symptoms of disease return when a patient has a relapse. Exacerbation is an increase in the severity of a disease or any of its symptoms.

FIGURE 4–11

Total hip joint and total knee joint replacement. A, Total hip joint replacement. A cementless prosthesis allows porous ingrowth of bone. **B,** Total knee joint replacement using a tibial metal retainer and a femoral component. The femoral component is chosen individually for each person according to the amount of healthy bone present.

4

		remission _____

Symptoms of disease lessen when the disease goes into remission.

resection _____

retro-	back, behind	retroperitoneal _____

The kidneys and adrenal glands are retroperitoneal organs.

sub-	under, less than	subcostal _____

subcutaneous _____

subtotal _____

A subtotal gastrectomy is a partial resection of the stomach.

subscapular _____

The scapula is the shoulder bone. Figure 4-12 shows its location.

syn-	with, together	syndrome _____

-DROME means to run or occur. Syndromes are groups of symptoms or signs of illness that occur together. Table 4-4 gives examples of syndromes.

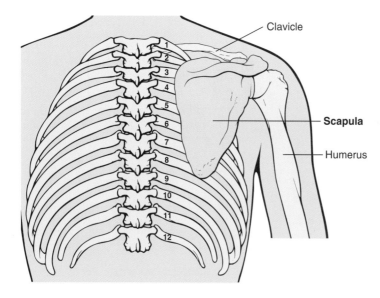

FIGURE 4–12

Scapula (shoulder bone), posterior view. The clavicle is the collar bone, and the humerus is the upper arm bone. (Modified from Chabner D-E: *The Language of Medicine,* ed 7, Philadelphia, 2004, WB Saunders.)

TABLE 4–4	SYNDROMES
acquired immunodeficiency syndrome (AIDS)	Symptoms are severe infections, malignancy (Kaposi sarcoma and lymphoma), fever, malaise (discomfort), and gastrointestinal disturbances. It is caused by a virus that damages lymphocytes (white blood cells).
Barlow syndrome (mitral valve prolapse)	Symptoms are abnormal sounds (murmurs) heard from the chest when listening with a stethoscope. These murmurs indicate that the mitral valve is not closing properly. Chest pain, dyspnea (difficult breathing), and fatigue are other symptoms.
carpal tunnel syndrome	Symptoms are pain, tingling, burning, and numbness of the hand. A nerve leading to the hand is compressed by connective tissue fibers in the wrist.
Down syndrome	Symptoms include mental retardation, flat face with a short nose, slanted eyes, broad hands and feet, stubby fingers, and protruding lower lip. The syndrome occurs when an extra chromosome is present in each cell of the body.
toxic shock syndrome	Symptoms are high fever, vomiting, diarrhea, rash, hypotension (low blood pressure), and shock. It is caused by a bacterial infection in the vagina of menstruating women using superabsorbent tampons.

tachy-	fast	tachycardia _____
		tachypnea _____
trans-	across, through	transabdominal _____
		transurethral _____

A ***transurethral resection*** of the prostate gland *is a* TURP. *Pieces of the prostate gland are removed through the urethra to relieve benign prostatic hypertrophy.*

| **tri-** | three | tricuspid valve _____ |

-CUSPID *means "pointed end," as of a spear. The tricuspid valve is on the right side of the heart. The mitral (bicuspid) valve is on the left side of the heart. Figure 4-13 shows the location of both valves and indicates the pathway of blood through the heart.*

| **ultra-** | beyond | ultrasonography _____ |

Figure 4-14 shows an ultrasonogram (sonogram) of a fetus.

| **uni-** | one | unilateral _____ |

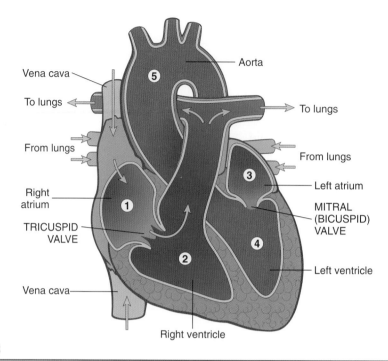

Vena cava

To lungs

From lungs

Aorta

To lungs

From lungs

Left atrium

MITRAL
(BICUSPID)
VALVE

Left ventricle

Right
atrium

TRICUSPID
VALVE

Vena cava

Right ventricle

FIGURE 4–13

Tricuspid and mitral valves of the heart. Blood enters the ***right atrium*** of the heart *(1)* from the big veins (venae cavae) and passes through the ***tricuspid valve*** to the ***right ventricle*** *(2)*. Blood then travels to the ***lungs*** where it loses carbon dioxide (a gaseous waste) and picks up oxygen. Blood returns to the heart into the ***left atrium*** *(3)* and passes through the mitral (bicuspid) valve to the ***left ventricle*** *(4)*. It is then pumped from the left ventricle out of the heart into the largest artery, the ***aorta*** *(5)*, which carries the blood to all parts of the body.

FIGURE 4–14

Ultrasonogram of my grandson Samuel August Thompson as a 19-week-old fetus. (Courtesy Dr. Elizabeth Chabner Thompson.)

IV. Exercises and Answers

Complete these exercises and check your answers. An important part of your success in learning medical terminology is checking your answers carefully in the answer key beginning on p. 145.

4

A. Give meanings for the following prefixes:

1. anti- _____

2. ana- _____

3. ad- _____

4. bi- _____

5. brady- _____

6. ab- _____

7. a-, an- _____

8. ante- _____

9. con- _____

10. dia- _____

B. Complete the following sentences with the medical terms below:

analysis	antigen	bradycardia
anemia	apnea	diarrhea
antibiotic	atrophy	
antibody	bilateral	

1. A patient with hearing loss in both ears has a(an) _____ condition.

2. Sudden infant death syndrome (SIDS) is an example of sleep _____.

3. A protein produced by white blood cells in response to a foreign substance, such as

   bacterium or virus, is a(an) _____.

4. A foreign substance, such as bacteria or virus, is a(an) _____.

5. Decrease in hemoglobin in the blood to below the normal range produces a

   condition known as _____.

6. A condition of frequent loose, watery stools that seem to "flow through" the body

   is called _____.

7. The separation of substances into their component parts is known as

_____.

8. An agent produced from molds or synthesized in a laboratory to destroy

microorganisms is a(an) _____.

9. A condition in which the heart rate is less than 60 beats per minute is

_____.

10. Having an arm in a cast and not using it can cause _____.

C. Give medical terms for the following meanings:

1. Without speech: _____

2. Lack of menstrual flow: _____

3. Before birth: _____

4. Glands located near the kidneys: _____ glands

5. An irregularity appearing with birth: _____ anomaly

6. Separation of waste materials from the blood when the kidneys fail:

_____

D. Give meanings for the following prefixes:

1. ec- _____   6. dys- _____

2. epi- _____   7. endo- _____

3. hemi- _____   8. ex- _____

4. hyper- _____   9. extra- _____

5. hypo- _____   10. in- _____

E. Complete the following sentences using the medical terms listed below:

dysmenorrhea   dysuria   extrahepatic
dysphagia   endoscopy   incision
dysplasia   epidermis
dyspnea   excision

1. Pain associated with menstrual flow is _____.

2. Cutting into a part of the body is a (an) _____.

3. Any abnormal development in tissues or organs is _____.

4. Cutting out of a part of the body is a (an) _____.

5. Painful burning sensation upon urination is _____.

6. Painful breathing that may be caused by anxiety, strenuous exercise, or certain

 heart conditions is _____.

7. The outer layer of skin is the _____.

8. Pertaining to outside the liver is _____.

9. Difficulty in swallowing is called _____.

10. Visual examination (via an endoscope) of what is within an organ is

 _____.

F. Complete the following medical terms from the meanings provided:

1. High blood pressure is _____tension.

2. A mass of blood above the membrane surrounding the brain is a(an)

 _____dural hemat_____.

3. A pregnancy that is out of place and usually located in a fallopian tube is a(an)

 _____topic pregnancy.

4. A condition of excessive (too much) blood sugar is _____emia.

5. A condition of deficient (too little) blood sugar is _____emia.

6. Glands that secrete hormones within the body are _____crine glands.

7. Increase in development (individual cells increase in size) often caused by overuse of a muscle or organ is hyper_____.

8. Paralysis of half of the body related to a stroke is _____plegia.

9. Excessive secretion of hormone from a gland in front of the trachea in the neck is hyper_____.

G. Give meanings for the following prefixes:

1. intra- _____

2. mal- _____

3. para- _____

4. peri- _____

5. poly- _____

6. inter- _____

7. meta- _____

8. neo- _____

9. post- _____

10. pre- _____

H. Give meanings for the following medical terms:

1. intervertebral _____

2. metastasis _____

3. metacarpals _____

4. intravenous _____

5. postmortem _____

6. periosteum _____

7. precancerous _____

8. neonatal _____

9. paraplegia _____

10. malignant _____

I. **Complete each of the sentences below by selecting from the following list of terms. The bolded words in each sentence should help you choose the correct term:**

adrenal glands   neoplasm   polyneuropathy
dyspnea   parathyroid glands   polyuria
extracranial   perianal   postpartum
intrauterine   polydipsia

1. An injury to the **outside** of the skull is a(an) _____ lesion.

2. Four small glands in the neck region **near** (posterior to) another endocrine gland

   are the _____.

3. Common symptoms of diabetes are **much** urination, or _____, and

   much thirst, or _____.

4. People suffering from asthma often have **difficult** breathing, which is called

   _____.

5. Bleeding can occur from cracks or sores **surrounding** the opening to the rectum.

   These are _____ fissures.

6. Two glands each located **near** (above) a kidney are _____.

7. A **new** growth, which can be malignant or benign, is a(an) _____.

8. Disease of **many** nerves is known as a(an) _____.

9. Any problem that affects the fetus **within** the womb is a(an) _____

   condition.

10. Women may experience moodiness and sad feelings **after** birth, a condition known

   as _____ depression.

J. Give meanings for the following prefixes:

1. pro- _____

2. quadri- _____

3. sub- _____

4. tachy- _____

5. trans- _____

6. uni- _____

7. re- _____

8. pros- _____

9. retro- _____

10. syn- _____

11. ultra- _____

12. tri- _____

K. Select from the following terms to complete each of the sentences below:

prolapse	remission	tachypnea
prosthesis	resection	tricuspid
quadriplegia	subtotal	ultrasonography
relapse	syndrome	unilateral

1. Removal or cutting out of an organ is a(an) _____.

2. Test that shows the structure of organs using sound waves beyond the normal

    range of hearing is _____.

3. An artificial part of the body is a(an) _____.

4. Recurrence of symptoms of an illness is a(an) _____.

5. Recovery and disappearance of symptoms is a(an) _____.

6. Rapid breathing is _____.

7. If the spinal cord is severed in the cervical region, paralysis of all four limbs,

    known as _____, occurs.

8. The _____ valve has three parts and is on the right side of the heart,

    between the upper and lower chambers.

9. If a patient has a(an) _____ gastrectomy, less than the complete

    stomach is removed.

10. Pain, tingling, burning, and numbness of the hand are symptoms of carpal tunnel

    _____.

L. Define the following terms that describe parts of the body:

1. subscapular _____

2. transabdominal _____

3. retroperitoneal _____

4. subcutaneous _____

5. intervertebral _____

M. Select from the following terms to complete the sentences below:

anemia   prolapse   tachycardia
aphasia   relapse   transurethral
paralysis   remission

1. After her ninth child, muscles in Ms. Smith's uterine wall weakened, causing her

   uterus to fall and _____ through her vagina.

2. After Mr. Jones' heart attack, his cardiologist noticed a rapid heart rhythm, or

   _____.

3. A CVA on the left side of the brain can cause a loss of speech, or _____.

4. Menorrhagia and lack of iron in Sharon's diet led to a condition of low hemoglobin

   and iron-deficiency _____.

5. The operation to remove part of Bill's enlarged (hypertrophied) prostate gland

   involved placing a catheter through his urethra and removing pieces of his prostate

   gland. The surgery, called a TURP, or _____ resection of the prostate

   gland, improved his ability to urinate. The prostate gland is at the base of the

   urinary bladder in males (see Figure 4-15).

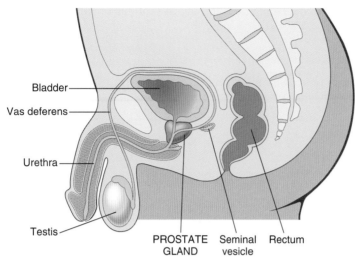

FIGURE 4–15

Prostate gland.

Bladder

Vas deferens

Urethra

Testis

PROSTATE Seminal Rectum
GLAND vesicle

N. Circle the correct meaning in each of the following:

1. Dys- and mal- both mean (outside, good, bad).

2. Hypo- and sub- both mean (under, above, outside).

3. Epi- and hyper- both mean (inside, beneath, above).

4. Con- and syn- both mean (apart, near, with).

5. Ultra- and meta- both mean (new, beyond, without).

6. Ante-, pre-, and pro- all mean (before, surrounding, between).

7. Ec- and extra- both mean (within, many, outside).

8. Endo-, intra-, and in- all mean (painful, within, through).

9. Post-, re-, and retro- all mean (behind, slow, together).

10. Uni- means (one, two, three).

11. Tri- means (one, two, three).

12. Bi- means (one, two, three).

O. Circle the term that best completes the meaning of the sentences in the following medical vignettes:

4

1. As part of her (**intravenous, postpartum, prenatal**) care, Bea underwent (**ultrasonography, endoscopy, urinalysis**) to determine the age, size, and development of her fetus.

2. Ellen's pregnancy test was positive, but she had excruciating pelvic pain. After an examination and ultrasound, the doctors diagnosed a(an) (**epidural, ectopic, subscapular**) pregnancy. She then underwent emergency surgery to remove the early pregnancy from the fallopian tube.

3. After noticing a suspicious-looking mole on her upper arm, Carole was diagnosed with (**malignant, benign, subtotal**) melanoma. This type of skin cancer is a(an) (**intrauterine, extrahepatic, neoplastic**) process and has a high likelihood of (**paralysis, dysplasia, metastasis**) to other areas of the body.

4. Carole's daughter, Annabelle, found a mole on her back and quickly had it checked out by her physician. Fortunately, after a biopsy, the pathology revealed a (**transabdominal, precancerous, perianal**) nevus (mole) that was considered (**chronic, unilateral, benign**). In the future, Annabelle will need close follow-up for other suspicious lesions.

5. Milton's blood pressure was 160/110. Normal blood pressure is 120/80. Because of his (**bradycardia, hypertension, dyspnea**), Milton's physician prescribed medication to reduce his risk of stroke.

Answers to Exercises

A

1. against	5. slow	8. before, forward
2. up, apart	6. away from	9. with, together
3. toward, near	7. no, not, without	10. through, complete
4. two, both		

B

1. bilateral	5. anemia	8. antibiotic
2. apnea	6. diarrhea	9. bradycardia
3. antibody	7. analysis	10. atrophy
4. antigen		

C

1. aphasia	3. antepartum, or prenatal	5. congenital
2. amenorrhea	4. adrenal	6. dialysis

4

D

1. out, outside
2. above, upon
3. half
4. excessive, too much, above
5. deficient, too little, below
6. bad, painful, difficult, abnormal
7. within, in, inner
8. out
9. outside of
10. in, into

E

1. dysmenorrhea
2. incision
3. dysplasia
4. excision
5. dysuria
6. dyspnea
7. epidermis
8. extrahepatic
9. dysphagia
10. endoscopy

F

1. **hyper**tension
2. **epi**dural hemat**oma**
3. **ect**opic
4. **hyperglyc**emia
5. **hypoglyc**emia
6. **endo**crine
7. hyper**trophy**
8. **hemi**plegia
9. hyper**thyroidism**

G

1. within
2. bad
3. beside, near, along the side of
4. surrounding
5. many, much
6. between
7. change, beyond
8. new
9. after, behind
10. before

H

1. pertaining to between the vertebrae (backbones)
2. change of place or beyond control (spread of a cancerous tumor to a secondary location)
3. beyond the wrist bones (carpals); hand bones
4. pertaining to within a vein
5. after death
6. membrane surrounding a bone
7. pertaining to a condition that comes before a malignancy; for example, dysplastic nevi (moles) that precede malignant melanoma
8. pertaining to before birth; a neonate is a newborn
9. condition of paralysis of the lower half of the body
10. cancerous; not benign

I

1. extracranial
2. parathyroid glands
3. polyuria; polydipsia
4. dyspnea
5. perianal
6. adrenal glands
7. neoplasm
8. polyneuropathy
9. intrauterine
10. postpartum

J

1. before, forward
2. four
3. under, less than
4. fast
5. across, through
6. one
7. back, behind
8. before, forward
9. back, behind
10. with, together
11. beyond
12. three

K

1. resection
2. ultrasonography
3. prosthesis; literally meaning "to put forward"

4. relapse
5. remission
6. tachypnea
7. quadriplegia
8. tricuspid

9. subtotal
10. syndrome

L

1. pertaining to under the scapula (shoulder bone)
2. pertaining to across or through the abdomen

3. pertaining to behind the peritoneum
4. pertaining to under the skin
5. pertaining to between the vertebrae (backbones)

M

1. prolapse   2. tachycardia   3. aphasia   4. anemia   5. transurethral

N

1. bad
2. under

3. above
4. with

5. beyond
6. before

7. outside
8. within

9. behind
10. one

11. three
12. two

O

1. prenatal, ultrasonography
2. ectopic
3. malignant, neoplastic, metastasis

4. precancerous, benign
5. hypertension

V. Review

Write the meaning of each of the following word parts, and remember to check your answers with the answer key on p. 150.

Prefixes

Prefix	Meaning	Prefix	Meaning
1. a-, an- _____		5. ante- _____	
2. ab- _____		6. anti- _____	
3. ad- _____		7. bi- _____	
4. ana- _____		8. brady- _____	

9. con-_____

10. dia-_____

11. dys-_____

12. ec-_____

13. endo-_____

14. epi-_____

15. ex-, extra-_____

16. hemi-_____

17. hyper-_____

18. hypo-_____

19. in-_____

20. inter-_____

21. intra-_____

22. mal-_____

23. meta-_____

24. neo-_____

25. para-_____

26. peri-_____

27. post-_____

28. pre-_____

29. pro-, pros-_____

30. quadri-_____

31. re-, retro-_____

32. sub-_____

33. syn-_____

34. tachy-_____

35. trans-_____

36. tri-_____

37. ultra-_____

38. uni-_____

Combining Forms

Combining Form	Meaning	Combining Form	Meaning
1. abdomin/o_____		6. cis/o_____	
2. an/o_____		7. cost/o_____	
3. bi/o_____		8. crani/o_____	
4. cardi/o_____		9. cutane/o_____	
5. carp/o_____		10. dur/o_____	

4

11. gen/o _____

12. glyc/o _____

13. hemat/o _____

14. later/o _____

15. nat/i _____

16. neur/o _____

17. norm/o _____

18. oste/o _____

19. peritone/o _____

20. plas/o _____

21. ren/o _____

22. scapul/o _____

23. son/o _____

24. thyroid/o _____

25. top/o _____

26. troph/o _____

27. urethr/o _____

28. uter/o _____

29. ven/o _____

30. vertebr/o _____

Suffixes

Suffix	Meaning	Suffix	Meaning
1. -al		11. -ine	
2. -ation		12. -ism	
3. -cision		13. -lysis	
4. -crine		14. -mortem	
5. -dipsia		15. -oma	
6. -emia		16. -ous	
7. -gen		17. -partum	
8. -graphy		18. -pathy	
9. -ia		19. -plasm	
10. -ic		20. -pnea	

21. -rrhea_____

22. -scopy_____

23. -section _____

24. -stasis _____

25. -tension _____

26. -thesis_____

27. -tic_____

28. -um _____

29. -uria _____

30. -y _____

Answers to Review

Prefixes

1. no, not, without
2. away from
3. toward
4. up, apart
5. before, forward
6. against
7. two
8. slow
9. with, together
10. through, complete
11. bad, painful, difficult, abnormal
12. out, outside
13. within, in, inner
14. above, upon
15. out, outside
16. half
17. excessive, above
18. below, under
19. in, into
20. between
21. within
22. bad
23. change, beyond
24. new
25. beside, near, along the side of
26. surrounding
27. after, behind
28. before
29. before, forward
30. four
31. back, behind
32. under, less than
33. with, together
34. fast
35. across, through
36. three
37. beyond
38. one

Combining Forms

1. abdomen
2. anus
3. life
4. heart
5. wrist bones
6. to cut
7. ribs
8. skull
9. skin
10. dura mater
11. to produce
12. sugar
13. blood
14. side
15. birth
16. nerve
17. rule, order
18. bone
19. peritoneum
20. formation, growth
21. kidney
22. shoulder blade (bone)
23. sound
24. thyroid gland
25. to put, place
26. development, nourishment
27. urethra
28. uterus
29. vein
30. vertebra (backbone)

Suffixes

1. pertaining to
2. process, condition
3. process of cutting
4. secretion
5. condition of thirst
6. blood condition
7. to produce
8. process of recording
9. condition, process
10. pertaining to
11. pertaining to
12. condition, process
13. loosening, breakdown, separation, destruction
14. death
15. tumor
16. pertaining to
17. birth
18. disease condition
19. formation
20. breathing
21. flow, discharge
22. process of visual examination
23. incision
24. to stand, place, stop, control
25. pressure
26. to put, place
27. pertaining to
28. structure
29. urine condition
30. process, condition

VI. Pronunciation of Terms

The terms that you have learned in this chapter are presented here with their pronunciations. The capitalized letters in boldface are the accented syllable. Pronounce each word out loud, then write its meaning in the space provided. All terms are defined in the *Glossary of Medical Terms,* p. 313.

Term	Pronunciation	Meaning
abnormal	ab-**NOR**-mal	
adrenal glands	ah-**DRE**-nal glanz	
analysis	ah-**NAL**-ih-sis	
anemia	ah-**NE**-me-ah	
antepartum	**AN**-te **PAR**-tum	
antibiotic	an-tih-bi-**OT**-ik	
antibody	**AN**-tih-bod-e	
antigen	**AN**-tih-jen	
aphasia	a-**FA**-ze-ah	
apnea	**AP**-ne-ah	
atrophy	**AT**-ro-fe	

4

benign	be-**NIN** _____
bilateral	bi-**LAT**-er-al _____
bradycardia	bra-de-**KAR**-de-ah _____
congenital anomaly	kon-**JEN**-ih-tal ah-**NOM**-ah-le _____
dialysis	di-**AL**-ih-sis _____
diarrhea	di-ah-**RE**-ah _____
dysphagia	dis-**FA**-jah _____
dysplasia	dis-**PLA**-zhah _____
dyspnea	**DISP**-ne-ah or disp-**NE**-ah _____
dysuria	dis-**U**-re-ah _____
ectopic pregnancy	ek-**TOP**-ik **PREG**-nan-se _____
endocrine glands	**EN**-do-krin glanz _____
endoscopy	en-**DOS**-ko-pe _____
epidural hematoma	ep-ih-**DUR**-al he-mah-**TO**-mah _____
excision	ek-**SIZH**-un _____
extrahepatic	eks-tra-heh-**PAT**-ik _____
hemigastrectomy	heh-me-gast-**REK**-to-me _____
hemiplegia	heh-me-**PLE**-jah _____
hyperglycemia	hi-per-gli-**SE**-me-ah _____
hypertension	hi-per-**TEN**-shun _____
hyperthyroidism	hi-per-**THI**-royd-izm _____
hypertrophy	hi-**PER**-tro-fe _____
hypoglycemia	hi-po-gli-**SE**-me-ah _____

incision	in-**SIZH**-un _____
intervertebral	in-ter-**VER**-teh-bral _____
intrauterine	in-trah-**U**-ter-in _____
intravenous	in-trah-**VE**-nus _____
malignant	mah-**LIG**-nant _____
metacarpal	met-ah-**KAR**-pal _____
metastasis	meh-**TAS**-tah-sis _____
neonatal	ne-o-**NA**-tal _____
neoplastic	ne-o-**PLAS**-tik _____
paralysis	pah-**RAL**-ih-sis _____
paraplegia	par-ah-**PLE**-jah _____
parathyroid glands	par-ah-**THI**-royd glanz _____
perianal	per-e-**A**-nal _____
periosteum	per-e-**OS**-te-um _____
polydipsia	pol-e-**DIP**-se-ah _____
polyneuropathy	pol-e-nu-**ROP**-ah-the _____
polyuria	pol-e-**UR**-e-ah _____
postmortem	post-**MOR**-tem _____
postpartum	post-**PAR**-tum _____
precancerous	pre-**KAN**-ser-us _____
prolapse	pro-**LAPS** _____
prosthesis	pros-**THE**-sis _____
quadriplegia	quah-drah-**PLE**-jah _____

4

relapse	re-**LAPS**
remission	re-**MISH**-un
resection	re-**SEK**-shun
retroperitoneal	reh-tro-peri-ih-to-**NE**-al
subcostal	sub-**KOS**-tal
subcutaneous	sub-ku-**TA**-ne-us
subdural hematoma	sub-**DUR**-al he-mah-**TO**-mah
subscapular	sub-**SKAP**-u-lar
subtotal	sub-**TO**-tal
syndrome	**SIN**-drom
tachycardia	tak-eh-**KAR**-de-ah
tachypnea	tak-ip-**NE**-ah
transabdominal	trans-ab-**DOM**-ih-nal
transurethral	trans-u-**RE**-thral
tricuspid valve	tri-**KUS**-pid valv
ultrasonography	ul-trah-son-**OG**-rah-fe
unilateral	u-nih-**LAT**-er-al
urinalysis	u-rih-**NAL**-ih-sis

VII. Practical Applications

Answers are found on p. 156.

A. Match the abnormal condition in Column I with the organ lesion or body part in Column II that may be the cause of the condition:

Column I Abnormal Condition		Column II Organ Lesion or Body Part
1. aphasia	_____	A. urinary bladder
2. dysphagia	_____	B. colon
3. diarrhea	_____	C. uterine cervix
4. quadriplegia	_____	D. left-sided brain lesion
5. hyperglycemia	_____	E. pancreas
6. dysuria	_____	F. lungs
7. paraplegia	_____	G. heart
8. bradycardia	_____	H. cervical spinal cord lesion
9. dyspnea	_____	I. esophagus
10. dysplasia	_____	J. lumbar spinal cord lesion

B. Pathology: Disease description—HYPERTHYROIDISM
   From the following terms complete the sentences in the paragraphs below:

antibiotics	exophthalmos	hypoplastic
antibodies	goiter	hyposecretion
bradycardia	hyperplastic	neoplastic
dyspnea	hypersecretion	tachycardia

1. Hyperthyroidism, also known as thyrotoxicosis or Graves disease, is marked by an

   excess of thyroid hormones. There is much evidence to support a hereditary factor

   in the development of this condition, and some consider it an autoimmune disorder

   caused by _____ that bind to the surface of thyroid gland cells and

   stimulate _____ of hormones (T_3 and T_4— triiodothyronine and

   thyroxine). The enlarged gland, histologically, is composed of _____

   follicles lined with hyperactive cells.

2. Symptoms of hyperthyroidism include restlessness, insomnia, weight loss,

   sweating, and rapid heartbeat, or _____. Abnormal protrusion of the

   eyes, known as _____, is another symptom. The patient also has an

   enlarged thyroid gland, called a(an) _____.

Answers to Practical Applications

A

1. D	3. B	5. E	7. J	9. F
2. I	4. H	6. A	8. G	10. C

B

1. antibodies, hypersecretion, hyperplastic   2. tachycardia, exophthalmos, goiter

VII. Picture Show

Answer the questions that follow each image. Correct answers are found on p. 159.

(Modified from Thibodeau GA, Patton KT: *Anatomy and Physiology,* ed 5, St Louis, 2003, Mosby.)

1. The arrows are pointing to muscles that lie between the ribs. They are the

    a. intracostal muscles   c. perianal muscles
    b. intercostal muscles   d. intrauterine muscles

(From Zitelli BJ, Davis HW: *Atlas of Pediatric Physical Diagnosis,* ed 4, St Louis, 2002, Mosby.)

1. This image shows the hand of an infant with (hint: the combining form for fingers is dactyl/o)

    a. syndactyly   c. transdactyly
    b. condactyly   d. polydactyly

2. This condition occurs as a(an):

    a. neoplastic anomaly   c. hypertensive anomaly
    b. congenital anomaly   d. ectopic pregnancy

4

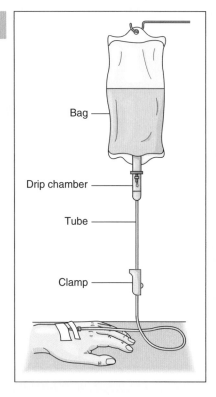

C

Bag

Drip chamber

Tube

Clamp

(Modified from Sorrentino SA: *Mosby's Textbook for Nursing Assistants,* ed 5, St Louis, 2000, Mosby.)

1. This equipment permits nutrients to enter the bloodstream and is used for:

      a. hemodialysis   c. intravenous feeding
      b. intrauterine feeding   d. peritoneal dialysis

2. Which term describes a condition or procedure that would likely make this equipment necessary?

      a. metacarpalgia   d. epidural hematoma
      b. hemigastrectomy   e. ultrasonography
      c. polyneuropathy

Answers to Picture Show

A

1. b

B

1. d   2. b

C

1. c   2. b

4

IX. Medical Scramble

Unscramble the letters to form a medical term from the clues. Use the letters in squares to complete the bonus term. Answers are upside down at the bottom of the page.

1. Harmless, not cancerous

___ ___ ☐ ___ ☐ ___ I N G B N E

2. Painful urination

___ ___ ___ ___ ___ ☐ ___ S Y R A D I U

3. Pertaining to a new born

☐ ___ ___ ___ ___ ___ ___ ___ L E O A T N A N

4. Condition associated with SIDS (sudden infant death syndrome)

___ ___ ___ ☐ ___ N E A A P

5. Organs shrink in size

☐ ☐ ___ ___ ___ ___ ___ P Y A R T O H

BONUS TERM: FOREIGN PROTEIN THAT CAUSES AN IMMUNE RESPONSE (hint: this protein is often part of bacteria and viruses and evokes production of antibodies)

☐ ☐ ☐ ☐ ☐ ☐ ☐

5

Medical Specialists and Case Reports

Chapter Sections

Chapter Objectives

- To describe the training process of physicians
- To identify medical specialists and describe their specialties
- To identify combining forms used in terms that describe specialists
- To decipher medical terminology as written in case reports

I. Introduction

This chapter reviews many of the terms you have learned in previous chapters and adds others related to medical specialists. In Section II, the training of physicians is described and specialists are listed with their specialties. Section III uses combining forms, which are found in the terms describing specialists, with familiar suffixes to test your knowledge of terms. In Section IV, short case reports are presented to illustrate the use of the medical language in context. As you read these reports, you will be impressed with your ability to understand medical terminology!

II. Medical Specialists

Doctors complete 4 years of medical school and then pass National Medical Board Examinations to receive an MD (Medical Doctor) degree. They may then begin postgraduate training, the length of which is at least 3 years and in some cases longer. This postgraduate training is known as *residency training*. Examples of residency programs are:

Anesthesiology	Administration of agents capable of bringing about a loss of sensation
Dermatology	Diagnosis and treatment of skin disorders
Emergency medicine	Care of patients that requires sudden and immediate action
Family practice	Primary care of all members of the family on a continuing basis
Internal medicine	Diagnosis of disorders and treatment with drugs
Ophthalmology	Diagnosis and treatment of eye disorders
Pathology	Diagnosis of the cause and nature of disease
Pediatrics	Diagnosis and treatment of children's disorders
Psychiatry	Diagnosis and treatment of disorders of the mind
Radiology	Diagnosis using x-rays and other procedures (ultrasound and magnetic resonance imaging)
Surgery	Treatment by manual (SURG- means hand) or operative methods

Examinations are administered after the completion of each residency program to certify the doctor's competency in that specialty area.

A physician may then choose to specialize further by doing *fellowship training*. Fellowships (lasting 2 to 5 years) train doctors in *clinical* (patient care) and *research* (laboratory) skills. For example, an *internist* (specialist in internal medicine) may choose fellowship training in internal medicine specialties such as neurology, nephrology, endocrinology, and oncology. A surgeon interested in further specialization may do fellowship training in thoracic surgery, neurosurgery, or plastic surgery. On completion of training and examinations, the doctor is then recognized as a specialist in that specialty area.

Medical specialists and an explanation of their specialties are listed below:

Medical Specialist	Specialty
allergist	Treatment of hypersensitivity reactions
anesthesiologist	Administration of agents for loss of sensation
cardiologist	Treatment of heart disease
cardiovascular surgeon	Surgery on the heart and blood vessels
colorectal surgeon	Surgery on the colon and rectum
dermatologist	Treatment of skin disorders
emergency practitioner	Immediate evaluation and treatment of people with acute injury and illness in a hospital setting
endocrinologist	Treatment of endocrine gland disorders
family practitioner	Primary care and treatment of families on a continuing basis
gastroenterologist	Treatment of stomach and intestinal disorders
geriatrician	Treatment of diseases of old age
gynecologist	Surgery and treatment of the female reproductive system
hematologist	Treatment of blood disorders
infectious disease specialist	Treatment of diseases caused by microorganisms
internist	Comprehensive care to adults in an office or hospital
nephrologist	Treatment of kidney diseases
neurologist	Treatment of nerve disorders
neurosurgeon	Surgery on the brain, spinal cord, and nerves
obstetrician	Treatment of pregnant women; delivery of babies
oncologist	Diagnosis and medical treatment of malignant and benign tumors
ophthalmologist	Surgical and medical treatment of eye disorders
orthopedist	Surgical treatment of bones, muscles, and joints
otolaryngologist	Treatment of the ear, nose, and throat
pathologist	Diagnosis of disease by analysis of cells
pediatrician	Treatment of diseases of children
physical medicine and rehabilitation specialist	Treatment to restore function after illness
psychiatrist	Treatment of mental disorders
pulmonary specialist	Treatment of lung diseases
radiologist	Examination of x-rays to determine a diagnosis; includes interpretation of ultrasound images and MRI and nuclear medicine as well
radiation oncologist	Treatment of disease with high-energy radiation
rheumatologist	Treatment of joint and muscle disorders
thoracic surgeon	Surgery on chest organs
urologist	Surgery on the urinary tract

5

III. Combining Forms and Vocabulary

The combining forms listed below should be familiar because they are found in the list of terms describing medical specialists. A medical term is included to illustrate the use of the combining form. Write the meaning of the medical term in the space provided. You can always check your answers with the *Glossary of Medical Terms* at the end of the book.

Combining Form	Meaning	Medical Term	Meaning
cardi/o	heart	cardiomegaly	_____
col/o	colon	colostomy	_____
dermat/o	skin	dermatitis	_____
endocrin/o	endocrine glands	endocrinology	_____
enter/o	intestines	enteritis	_____
esthesi/o	sensation	anesthesiology	_____
gastr/o	stomach	gastroscopy	_____
ger/o	old age	geriatrics	_____
gynec/o	woman, female	gynecology	_____
hemat/o	blood	hematoma	_____
iatr/o	treatment	iatrogenic	_____
		IATR/O- *means treatment by a physician or with medicines. An iatrogenic illness is* produced (-GENIC) *unexpectedly by a treatment.*	
laryng/o	voice box	laryngeal	_____
lymph/o	lymph	lymphadenopathy	_____
		Lymph "glands" are actually lymph nodes, located all over the body but especially in **axillary** *(armpit),* **inguinal** *(groin),* **cervical** *(neck), and* **mediastinal** *(area between the lungs) regions. Lymphadenopathy often refers to the presence of malignant cells in lymph nodes.*	

nephr/o	kidney	nephrostomy _____
		A catheter (tube) is inserted into the kidney for drainage of fluid.
neur/o	nerve	neuralgia _____
nos/o	disease	nosocomial _____
		A nosocomial infection is acquired during hospitalization (COMI/O- means to care for).
obstetr/o	midwife	obstetric _____
onc/o	tumor	oncogenic _____
		Oncogenic viruses give rise to tumors.
ophthalm/o	eye	ophthalmologist _____
opt/o	eye	optometrist _____
		An optometrist examines (METR/O- means to measure) eyes and prescribes glasses but cannot treat eye diseases.
optic/o	eye	optician _____
		Opticians grind lenses and fit glasses but do not examine eyes, prescribe glasses, or treat eye diseases.
orth/o	straight	orthopedist _____
		PED/O- comes from the Greek, paidos, *meaning "child." In the past, orthopedists were concerned with straightening bone deformities in children. Now, they treat bone, muscle, and joint disorders in adults as well.*
ot/o	ear	otitis _____
path/o	disease	pathology _____
ped/o	child	pediatrics _____
psych/o	mind	psychosis _____
pulmon/o	lung	pulmonary _____

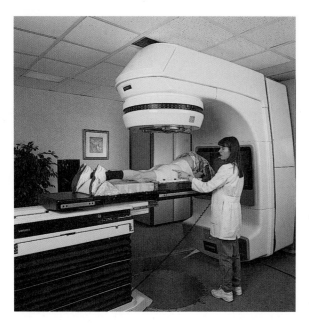

FIGURE 5–1

Radiation therapy. The patient is positioned under a radiation therapy machine (linear accelerator) to receive treatment for a lesion in the posterior portion of his hip. (Courtesy Dr. Arthur Brimberg, Riverhill Radiation Oncology, Yonkers, NY.)

| **radi/o** | x-rays | radiotherapy _____ |

Radiotherapy is also called radiation therapy. *See Figure 5-1.*

| **rect/o** | rectum | rectocele _____ |

-CELE *means a hernia or protrusion. The walls of the rectum weaken and bulge forward toward the vagina. See Figure 5-2.*

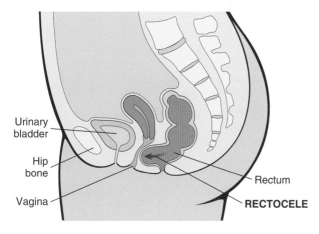

Urinary bladder

Hip bone

Vagina

Rectum

RECTOCELE

FIGURE 5–2

Rectocele. (Modified from Chabner D-E: *The Language of Medicine,* ed 7, Philadelphia, 2004, WB Saunders.)

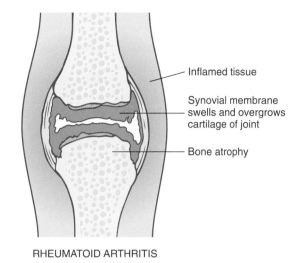

Bone

Cartilage

Joint space

Synovial membrane

Bone

Inflamed tissue

Synovial membrane swells and overgrows cartilage of joint

Bone atrophy

NORMAL JOINT   RHEUMATOID ARTHRITIS

FIGURE 5–3

Normal joint and joint with rheumatoid arthritis.

rheumat/o	flow, fluid	rheumatology _____

Joints can fill with fluid when diseased, hence RHEUMAT/O- indicates a problem with a swollen joint. Rheumatoid arthritis is a chronic inflammatory disease of joints and connective tissues that leads to deformation of joints. See Figures 5-3 and 5-4.

rhin/o	nose	rhinorrhea _____
thorac/o	chest	thoracotomy _____
ur/o	urinary tract	urology _____
vascul/o	blood vessels	vasculitis _____

FIGURE 5–4

Advanced rheumatoid arthritis of the hands. Notice the soft tissue swelling and deformed joints—fingers, knuckles, and wrist. Atrophy of muscles and tendons (connecting muscles to bones) causes one joint surface to slip past the other (subluxation). (From Lewis SM, Heitkemper MM, Dirksen SR: *Medical-Surgical Nursing: Assessment and Management of Clinical Problems,* ed 6, St Louis, Mosby, 2004.)

IV. Case Reports

Here are short case reports related to medical specialties. Many of the terms are
familiar; others are explained in the *Glossary of Medical Terms* on p. 313. For every
case, write the meaning of the boldface term in the space provided.

CASE 1 · **CARDIOLOGY**

Mr. Rose was admitted to the Cardiac Care Unit (CCU) after a severe **myocardial
infarction**. Previously, he had suffered from **angina** (due to **ischemia**) and **hypertension**.
He is being treated with **antiarrhythmic** drugs, **diuretics,** and **anticoagulants**. If his
recovery proceeds as expected, he will be discharged in 3 weeks.

angina _____

antiarrhythmic _____

anticoagulant _____

diuretic _____

hypertension _____

ischemia _____

myocardial infarction _____

CASE 2 · **GYNECOLOGY**

Ms. Sessions has had **dysmenorrhea** and **menorrhagia** for several months. She is also **anemic.** Because of the presence of large **fibroids,** as seen on a pelvic **ultrasound** exam **(sonogram),** a **hysterectomy** is recommended. After it was removed, the uterus was opened to reveal fibroids **(leiomyomas)** bulging into the uterine cavity and displaying a firm, white appearance. See Figure 5-5.

FIGURE 5–5

Fibroids (leiomyomas). These are benign tumors of the uterus. (From Cotran RS, Kumar V, Collins T: *Robbins Pathologic Basis of Disease,* ed 6, Philadelphia, 1999, WB Saunders.)

anemic _____

dysmenorrhea _____

fibroids _____

hysterectomy _____

leiomyomas _____

menorrhagia _____

sonogram _____

ultrasound _____

5

CASE 3 · **ONCOLOGY**

The patient is a 26-year-old female with a previous diagnosis of **mediastinal** and **intra-abdominal Hodgkin disease.** She was admitted to the hospital for abdominal **CT scan** and **percutaneous** liver **biopsy** after the discovery of possible recurrence of tumor. Following the assessment of her **platelet** count, a percutaneous liver biopsy was performed, showing normal **hepatic** tissue. The CT scan was normal as well. The patient was later scheduled for further evaluation and **peritoneoscopy** to assess possible **lymphadenopathy.**

biopsy _____

CT scan _____

hepatic _____

Hodgkin disease _____

intra-abdominal _____

lymphadenopathy _____

mediastinal _____

percutaneous _____

peritoneoscopy _____

platelet _____

CASE 4 · **UROLOGY**

Patty Smith has a history of lower back pain associated with **hematuria** and **dysuria**. She has an appointment at the hospital for investigation of her symptoms. Tests include an **intravenous pyelogram (IVP)** and **cystoscopy**. The findings of these tests confirmed the diagnosis of **renal calculus**. **Lithotripsy** was recommended, and her **prognosis** is favorable. Figure 5-6 shows a patient receiving lithotripsy to crush a renal calculus.

FIGURE 5–6

Lithotripsy.

X-ray (fluoroscope) probe

Lithotriptor

cystoscopy _____

dysuria _____

hematuria _____

intravenous pyelogram (IVP) _____

lithotripsy _____

prognosis _____

renal calculus _____

CASE 5 · **GASTROENTEROLOGY**

Mr. Pepper suffers from **dyspepsia** and sharp **abdominal** pain. A recent episode of **hematemesis** has left him very weak and **anemic**. **Gastroscopy** and **upper GI series** with **barium** revealed the presence of a large **ulcer**. Figure 5-7 shows a photograph of a peptic ulcer located in the stomach. Mr. Pepper will be admitted to the hospital and scheduled for a partial **gastrectomy**.

FIGURE 5–7

Peptic (gastric) ulcer. (From Lewis SM, Heitkemper MM, Dirksen SR: *Medical-Surgical Nursing: Assessment and Management of Clinical Problems,* ed 5, St Louis, 2004, Mosby.)

abdominal _____

anemic _____

barium _____

dyspepsia _____

gastrectomy _____

gastroscopy _____

hematemesis _____

ulcer _____

upper GI series _____

CASE 6 · **RADIOLOGY**

Examination: **Thoracic cavity.** PA **(posterior-anterior)** and **lateral** chest. There is a patchy **infiltrate** in the right lower **lobe** seen best in the lateral view. The heart and **mediastinal** structures are normal. No evidence of **pleural effusion.**

Impression: Right lower lobe **pneumonia**

anterior _____

infiltrate _____

lateral _____

lobe _____

mediastinal _____

pleural effusion _____

pneumonia _____

posterior _____

thoracic cavity _____

CASE 7 · ORTHOPEDICS

A 20-year-old male patient was admitted to the hospital following a motorcycle accident. In the accident he sustained **fractures** of the right **fibula** (see Figure 5-8, *A*), right **femur**, and **pelvis** and **intra-abdominal** injuries. He was taken to surgery, and internal **fixation** of the right femur was performed. A cast was applied for immobilization, and the fibula healed on its own with **callus** formation (Figure 5-8, *B*).

A   B

FIGURE 5–8

A, Fracture of the fibula. B, Callus formation, 6 weeks later. (Courtesy Dr. Barbara Weissman, Brigham and Women's Hospital, Boston, Mass. From Cotran RS, Kumar V, Collins T: *Robbins Pathologic Basis of Disease,* ed 6, Philadelphia, 1999, WB Saunders.)

callus _____

femur _____

fibula _____

fixation _____

fracture _____

intra-abdominal _____

pelvis _____

CASE 8 · **NEPHROLOGY**

A 52-year-old man with **chronic renal failure** secondary to long-standing **hypertension** has been maintained on **hemodialysis** for the past 18 months. For the past 3 weeks, during the dialysis sessions, he has become moderately **hypotensive,** with symptoms of dizziness. Consequently, we have decided to withhold his **antihypertensive** medications prior to dialysis.

antihypertensive _____

chronic _____

hemodialysis _____

hypertension _____

hypotensive _____

renal failure _____

CASE 9 · **ENDOCRINOLOGY**

A 36-year-old woman known to have **type I diabetes mellitus** was brought to the emergency room after being found collapsed in her home. She had experienced 3 days of extreme weakness, **polyuria,** and **polydipsia.** It was discovered that a few days prior to her admission she had discontinued her **insulin** in a suicide attempt.

insulin _____

polydipsia _____

polyuria _____

type I diabetes mellitus _____

5

CASE 10 · **NEUROLOGY**

Ms. Rose is admitted with severe, throbbing **unilateral frontal cephalgia** that has lasted for 2 days. Light makes her cringe, and she has **nausea**. Before the onset of these symptoms, she saw zigzag lines for about 20 minutes. Diagnosis is **acute migraine** with **aura**. A **vasoconstrictor** is prescribed, and Ms. Rose's condition is improving. (Migraine headaches are thought to be caused by sudden **dilation** of blood vessels.)

acute _____

aura _____

cephalgia _____

dilation _____

frontal _____

migraine _____

nausea _____

unilateral _____

vasoconstrictor _____

V. Exercises and Answers

Complete these exercises and check your answers. An important part of your success in learning medical terminology is checking your answers carefully in the answer key beginning on p. 183.

A. Match each of the following residency programs to its description below:

anesthesiology   internal medicine   psychiatry
dermatology   ophthalmology   radiology
emergency medicine   pathology   surgery
family practice   pediatrics

1. Treatment by operation or manual (hand) methods: _____

2. Diagnosis of adult disorders and treatment with drugs: _____

3. Diagnosis and treatment of disorders of the mind: _____

4. Primary care of all family members on a continuing basis: _____

5. Diagnosis and treatment of skin disorders: _____

6. Diagnosis and treatment of eye disorders: _____

7. Diagnosis of disease using x-rays: _____

8. Diagnosis and treatment of children's disorders: _____

9. Care of patients that requires immediate action: _____

10. Administration of agents that cause loss of sensation: _____

11. Diagnosis of disease by examining cells and tissues: _____

B. Name the doctor who treats the following problems (first letters are given):

1. kidney diseases   n _____

2. tumors   o _____

3. broken bones   o _____

4. female diseases   g _____

5. eye disorders   o _____

6. heart disorders   c _____

7. nerve disorders   n _____

8. lung disorders   p _____

9. mental disorders   p _____

10. stomach and intestinal disorders   g _____

C. Match the medical specialists in Column I to their specialties in Column II:

Column I		Column II
1. urologist	_____	A. operates on the large intestine
2. thoracic surgeon	_____	B. treats blood disorders
3. radiation oncologist	_____	C. treats thyroid and pituitary gland disorders
4. colorectal surgeon	_____	D. delivers babies
5. endocrinologist	_____	E. treats children and their disorders
6. obstetrician	_____	F. operates on the urinary tract
7. radiologist	_____	G. treats disorders of the skin
8. pediatrician	_____	H. treats tumors by using high-energy radiation
9. hematologist	_____	I. operates on the chest
10. dermatologist	_____	J. examines x-rays to diagnose disease

D. Complete each of the sentences below using a term from the following list:

clinical	oncologist	orthopedist
geriatrician	ophthalmologist	pathologist
infectious disease specialist	optician	research
	optometrist	surgeon

1. A doctor who diagnoses and treats diseases that are caused by microorganisms is a(an) _____.

2. A doctor who does bone surgery is a(an) _____.

3. A doctor who takes care of patients does _____ medicine.

4. A person who grinds lenses and fills prescriptions for eye glasses is a(an)

    _____.

5. A doctor who reads biopsy samples and performs autopsies is a(an)

    _____.

6. A doctor who treats cancerous tumors is a(an) _____.

7. A person who can examine eyes and prescribe eye glasses but cannot treat eye

    disorders is a(an) _____.

8. A doctor who operates on patients is a(an) _____.

9. A doctor who does experiments with test tubes and laboratory equipment is

    interested in _____ medicine.

10. A doctor who specializes in treatment of disorders of the eye is a(an)

    _____.

11. A doctor who specializes in the treatment of older people is a(an)

    _____.

E. Which medical specialist would you consult for the following medical conditions? The first letter of the specialist is given.

1. arthritis   r _____

2. otitis media   o _____

3. anemia   h _____

4. urinary bladder displacement   u _____

5. chronic bronchitis   p _____

6. cerebrovascular accident   n _____

7. breast cancer   o _____

8. coronary artery blockages   c _____
   (bypass surgery)

9. dislocated shoulder bone   o _____

10. thyroid gland enlargement   e _____

11. kidney disease   n _____

12. acne (skin disorder)   d _____

13. hay fever (hypersensitivity reaction)   a _____

14. viral and bacterial diseases   i _____

F. Give the meaning for each of the following medical terms:

1. neuralgia _____

2. pathology _____

3. cardiomegaly _____

4. nephrostomy _____

5. thoracotomy _____

6. laryngeal _____

7. otitis _____

8. colostomy _____

9. pulmonary _____

10. iatrogenic _____

11. gastroscopy _____

12. radiotherapy _____

13. anesthesiology _____

14. enteritis _____

15. nosocomial _____

G. Use the following combining forms and suffixes to make the medical terms called for:

Combining Forms		Suffixes	
aden/o	onc/o	-algia	-pathy
col/o	ophthalm/o	-ectomy	-scopy
laryng/o	ot/o	-genic	-stomy
lymph/o	path/o	-itis	-therapy
nephr/o	psych/o	-logy	-tomy
neur/o	thorac/o	-osis	

1. Inflammation of the ear: _____

2. Removal of a nerve: _____

3. Incision of the chest: _____

4. Study of tumors: _____

5. Pertaining to producing disease: _____

6. Inflammation of the voice box: _____

7. Opening of the large intestine to the outside of the body: _____

8. Visual examination of the eye: _____

9. Abnormal condition of the mind: _____

10. Inflammation of the kidney: _____

11. Removal of the large intestine: _____

12. Pain in the ear: _____

13. Treatment of the mind: _____

14. Pertaining to producing tumors: _____

15. Disease of lymph glands (nodes): _____

H. Circle the term that best completes the meaning of the sentences in the following medical vignettes:

1. Dr. Butler is a physician who operates on hearts. He trained as a **(neurologic, cardiovascular, pulmonary)** surgeon. Often, his procedures require that Dr. Smith, a(an) **(gynecologic, ophthalmic, thoracic)** surgeon, assist him when the chest and lungs need surgical intervention.

2. Pauline noticed a rash over most of her body. First she saw Dr. Cole, her **(family practitioner, oncologist, radiologist)** who performs her yearly physicals. Dr. Cole, who is not a(an) **(endocrinologist, orthopedist, dermatologist)** by training, referred her to a skin specialist to make the proper diagnosis and treat the rash.

3. Dr. Liu is a(an) **(internist, obstetrician, pediatrician)** as well as a(an) **(nephrologist, urologist, gynecologist)** and can take care of her female patients before, during, and after their pregnancies.

4. After her sixth pregnancy, Sally developed an abnormal condition at the lower end of her colon. She went to a(an) **(gastroenterologist, hematologist, optometrist)**, who made the diagnosis of protrusion of the rectum into the vagina. She then consulted colorectal and gynecologic surgeons to make an appropriate treatment plan for her condition, known as a **(vasculitis, rectocele, colostomy).**

5. In the cancer clinic, patients often must see a medical **(oncologist, orthopedist, rheumatologist),** who administers chemotherapy, and a(an) **(psychiatrist, radiation oncologist, radiologist),** who prescribes and supervises **(drugs, surgery, radiation therapy)** to treat tumors with high-energy protons and electrons.

FIGURE 5–9

Pedunculated polyp in the descending colon. It is arising from the mucosal surface of the colon and projecting into the lumen of the colon. (From Lewis SM, Heitkemper MM, Dirksen SR: *Medical-Surgical Nursing: Assessment and Management of Clinical Problems,* ed 5, St Louis, 2004, Mosby.)

6. While recovering from successful surgery in the hospital, Janet developed a cough and fever. Her surgeon ordered a chest x-ray and suspected a(an) **(oncogenic, nosocomial, iatrogenic)** pneumonia. A(an) **(anesthesiologist, neurologist, infectious disease specialist)** was called in to diagnose and treat the hospital-acquired disease condition.

7. Sam had noticed bright red rectal bleeding for several days when he finally saw his family practitioner. This physician referred him to a(an) **(endocrinologist, urologist, gastroenterologist)**. A **(laparoscopy, colonoscopy, bronchoscopy)** was scheduled, which revealed a large pedunculated (on a stalk) polyp (benign growth) in the descending colon. See Figure 5-9. The polyp was resected and sent to **(pathology, hematology, infectious disease)** for evaluation. Fortunately, it was a noncancerous or **(malignant, metastatic, benign)** lesion. Sam will need follow-up **(laparotomy, endoscopy, laparoscopy)** in a year.

Answers to Exercises

A

1. surgery
2. internal medicine
3. psychiatry
4. family practice
5. dermatology
6. ophthalmology
7. radiology
8. pediatrics
9. emergency medicine
10. anesthesiology
11. pathology

B

1. nephrologist
2. oncologist
3. orthopedist
4. gynecologist
5. ophthalmologist
6. cardiologist (internist) or cardiovascular surgeon (surgeon)
7. neurologist
8. pulmonary specialist
9. psychiatrist
10. gastroenterologist

5

C

1. F	3. H	5. C	7. J	9. B
2. I	4. A	6. D	8. E	10. G

D

1. infectious disease specialist
2. orthopedist
3. clinical
4. optician
5. pathologist
6. oncologist
7. optometrist
8. surgeon
9. research
10. ophthalmologist
11. geriatrician

E

1. rheumatologist
2. otolaryngologist
3. hematologist
4. urologist
5. pulmonary specialist
6. neurologist
7. oncologist
8. cardiovascular surgeon
9. orthopedist
10. endocrinologist
11. nephrologist
12. dermatologist
13. allergist
14. infectious disease specialist

F

1. nerve pain
2. study of disease
3. enlargement of the heart
4. opening from the kidney to the outside of the body
5. incision of the chest
6. pertaining to the voice box
7. inflammation of the ear
8. opening of the colon to the outside of the body
9. pertaining to the lungs
10. pertaining to an abnormal condition that is produced by treatment
11. process of visual examination of the stomach (using an endoscope)
12. treatment of disease using high-energy radiation
13. study of loss of sensation or feeling
14. inflammation of the intestines (usually small intestine)
15. pertaining to a disease acquired in the hospital

G

1. otitis
2. neurectomy
3. thoracotomy
4. oncology
5. pathogenic
6. laryngitis
7. colostomy
8. ophthalmoscopy
9. psychosis
10. nephritis
11. colectomy
12. otalgia
13. psychotherapy
14. oncogenic
15. lymphadenopathy

H

1. cardiovascular, thoracic
2. family practitioner, dermatologist
3. obstetrician, gynecologist
4. gastroenterologist, rectocele
5. oncologist, radiation oncologist, radiation therapy
6. nosocomial, infectious disease specialist
7. gastroenterologist, colonoscopy, pathology, benign, endoscopy

VI. Review

Test your understanding of the combining forms and suffixes in this chapter by completing this review. Remember to check your responses with the Answers to Review on p. 186.

Combining Forms

Combining Form	Meaning	Combining Form	Meaning
1. aden/o		18. obstetr/o	
2. cardi/o		19. onc/o	
3. col/o		20. ophthalm/o	
4. dermat/o		21. opt/o, optic/o	
5. endocrin/o		22. orth/o	
6. enter/o		23. ot/o	
7. esthesi/o		24. path/o	
8. gastr/o		25. ped/o	
9. ger/o		26. psych/o	
10. gynec/o		27. pulmon/o	
11. hemat/o		28. radi/o	
12. iatr/o		29. rect/o	
13. laryng/o		30. rheumat/o	
14. lymph/o		31. rhin/o	
15. nephr/o		32. thorac/o	
16. neur/o		33. ur/o	
17. nos/o		34. vascul/o	

Suffixes

Suffix	Meaning	Suffix	Meaning
1. -algia	_____	10. -oma	_____
2. -ary	_____	11. -osis	_____
3. -cele	_____	12. -pathy	_____
4. -eal	_____	13. -rrhea	_____
5. -genic	_____	14. -scopy	_____
6. -ist	_____	15. -stomy	_____
7. -itis	_____	16. -therapy	_____
8. -logy	_____	17. -tomy	_____
9. -megaly	_____		

Answers to Review

Combining Forms

1. gland	13. voice box	25. child
2. heart	14. lymph	26. mind
3. colon	15. kidney	27. lung
4. skin	16. nerve	28. x-rays
5. endocrine glands	17. disease	29. rectum
6. intestines	18. midwife	30. flow, fluid
7. sensation	19. tumor	31. nose
8. stomach	20. eye	32. chest
9. old age	21. eye	33. urinary tract
10. woman	22. straight	34. blood vessels
11. blood	23. ear	
12. treatment	24. disease	

Suffixes

1. pain	7. inflammation	13. flow
2. pertaining to	8. study of	14. process of visual examination
3. hernia, protrusion	9. enlargement	15. opening
4. pertaining to	10. mass, tumor	16. treatment
5. pertaining to producing	11. abnormal condition	17. incision
6. specialist	12. disease, emotion	

VII. Pronunciation of Terms

The terms that you have learned in this chapter are presented here with their pronunciations. The capitalized letters in boldface represent the accented syllable. Pronounce each word out loud, then write the meaning in the space provided.

Term	Pronunciation	Meaning
anesthesiology	an-es-the-ze-**OL**-o-je	_____
cardiologist	kar-de-**OL**-o-jist	_____
cardiovascular surgeon	kar-de-o-**VAS**-ku-lar **SUR**-jin	_____
clinical	**KLIN**-eh-kal	_____
colorectal surgeon	ko-lo-**REK**-tal **SUR**-jin	_____
colostomy	ko-**LOS**-to-me	_____
dermatologist	der-mah-**TOL**-o-jist	_____
dermatology	der-mah-**TOL**-o-je	_____
emergency medicine	e-**MER**-jen-se **MED**-ih-sin	_____
endocrinologist	en-do-krih-**NOL**-o-jist	_____
enteritis	en-teh-**RI**-tis	_____
family practitioner	**FAM**-ih-le prak-**TIH**-shan-er	_____
gastroenterologist	gas-tro-en-ter-**OL**-o-jist	_____
gastroscopy	gas-**TROS**-ko-pe	_____
geriatric	jer-e-**AH**-trik	_____
geriatrician	jer-e-ah-**TRISH**-shan	_____
gynecologist	gi-neh-**KOL**-o-jist	_____
gynecology	gi-neh-**KOL**-o-je	_____
hematologist	he-mah-**TOL**-o-jist	_____

hematoma	he-mah-**TO**-mah _____
iatrogenic	i-ah-tro-**JEN**-ik _____
infectious disease	in-**FEK**-shus dih-**ZEZ** _____
internal medicine	in-**TER**-nal **MED**-ih-sin _____
laryngitis	lah-rin-**JI**-tis _____
lymphadenopathy	limf-ah-deh-**NOP**-ah-the _____
nephrologist	neh-**FROL**-o-jist _____
nephrostomy	neh-**FROS**-to-me _____
neuralgia	nu-**RAL**-jah _____
neurologist	nu-**ROL**-o-jist _____
neurosurgeon	nu-ro-**SUR**-jin _____
nosocomial	nos-o-**KO**-me-al _____
obstetrician	ob-steh-**TRISH**-un _____
obstetrics	ob-**STET**-riks _____
oncogenic	ong-ko-**JEN**-ik _____
oncologist	ong-**KOL**-o-jist _____
ophthalmologist	of-thal-**MOL**-o-jist _____
ophthalmology	of-thal-**MOL**-o-je _____
optician	op-**TISH**-an _____
optometrist	op-**TOM**-eh-trist _____
orthopedist	or-tho-**PE**-dist _____
otitis	o-**TI**-tis _____

otolaryngologist	o-to-lah-rin-**GOL**-o-jist _____
pathologist	pah-**THOL**-o-jist _____
pathology	pah-**THOL**-o-je _____
pediatric	pe-de-**AT**-rik _____
pediatrician	pe-de-ah-**TRISH**-un _____
psychiatrist	si-**KI**-ah-trist _____
psychosis	si-**KO**-sis _____
pulmonary specialist	**PUL**-mo-ner-e **SPESH**-ah-list _____
radiation oncologist	ra-de-**A**-shun ong-**KOL**-o-jist _____
radiologist	ra-de-**OL**-o-jist _____
radiotherapy	ra-de-o-**THER**-ah-pe _____
rectocele	**REK**-to-sel _____
research	**RE**-surch _____
rheumatologist	roo-mah-**TOL**-o-jist _____
rheumatology	roo-mah-**TOL**-o-je _____
rhinorrhea	ri-no-**RE**-ah _____
surgery	**SUR**-jer-e _____
thoracic surgeon	tho-**RAS**-ik **SUR**-jin _____
thoracotomy	tho-rah-**KOT**-o-me _____
urologist	u-**ROL**-o-jist _____
vasculitis	vas-ku-**LI**-tis _____

5

VIII. Practical Applications

The exercises in this section are divided into three groups, each of which consists of a list of allied health specialists followed by a set of job descriptions. For each group, match each specialist to the appropriate job description and then check your answers with the answer key at the end of the Practical Applications section.

Group A

1. nurse anesthetist   _____

2. audiologist   _____

3. blood bank technologist   _____

4. chiropractor   _____

5. clinical laboratory technician _____

6. dental assistant   _____

7. dental hygienist   _____

8. dental laboratory technician   _____

9. diagnostic medical sonographer _____

10. dietitian/nutritionist   _____

    a. Treats patients with health problems associated with the muscular, nervous, and skeletal systems, especially the spine
    b. Prepares materials (crowns, bridges) for use by a dentist
    c. Works with people who have hearing problems by using testing devices to measure hearing loss
    d. Provides preventive dental care and teaches the practice of good oral hygiene
    e. Collects, types, and prepares blood and its components for transfusions
    f. Aids in the delivery of anesthesia during surgery
    g. Assists a dentist with dental procedures
    h. Performs diagnostic ultrasound procedures
    i. Plans nutrition programs and supervises the preparation and serving of meals
    j. Performs tests to examine and analyze body fluids, tissues, and cells

Group B

1. EKG technician _____

2. emergency medical technician/paramedic _____

3. health information management professional _____

4. home health aide _____

5. licensed practical nurse _____

6. medical assistant _____

7. medical laboratory technician _____

8. nuclear medicine technologist _____

9. nursing aide _____

10. occupational therapist _____

    a. Cares for elderly, disabled, and ill persons in their own homes, helping them live there instead of in an institution

    b. Performs routine tests and laboratory procedures

    c. Designs, manages, and administers the use of heath care data and information

    d. Operates an electrocardiograph to record EKGs, Holter monitoring, and stress tests

    e. Performs radioactive tests and procedures under the supervision of a nuclear medicine physician, who interprets the results

    f. Gives immediate care and transports sick or injured to medical facilities

    g. Helps physicians examine and treat patients and performs tasks to keep offices running smoothly

    h. Cares for the sick, injured, convalescing, and handicapped, under the direct supervision of physicians and registered nurses; provides basic bedside care

    i. Helps individuals with mentally, physically, developmentally, emotionally disabling conditions to develop, recover, or maintain daily living and working skills

    j. Helps care for physically or mentally ill, injured, or disabled patients confined to nursing, hospital, or residential care facilities; known as nursing assistants or hospital attendants

Group C

1. ophthalmic medical technician _____

2. phlebotomist _____

3. physical therapist _____

4. physician assistant _____

5. radiation therapist _____

6. radiographer/image technologist _____

7. registered nurse _____

8. respiratory therapist _____

9. speech language pathologist _____

10. surgical technologist _____

    a. Evaluates, treats, and cares for patients with breathing disorders
    b. Draws and tests blood under the supervision of a medical technologist or laboratory manager
    c. Cares for sick and injured people by assessing and recording symptoms, assisting physicians during treatments and examinations, and administering medications
    d. Prepares cancer patients for treatment and administers prescribed doses of ionizing radiation to specific areas of the body
    e. Helps ophthalmologists provide medical eye care
    f. Examines, diagnoses, and treats patients, under the direct supervision of a physician
    g. Assists in operations under the supervision of surgeons or registered nurses
    h. Improves the mobility, relieves the pain, and prevents or limits permanent physical disabilities of patients suffering from injuries or disease
    i. Produces x-ray images of parts of the body for use in diagnosing medical problems
    j. Assesses and treats persons with speech, language, voice, and fluency disorders

Answers to Practical Applications

Group A

| 1. f | 3. e | 5. j | 7. d | 9. h |
| 2. c | 4. a | 6. g | 8. b | 10. i |

Group B

| 1. d | 3. c | 5. h | 7. b | 9. j |
| 2. f | 4. a | 6. g | 8. e | 10. i |

Group C

| 1. e | 3. h | 5. d | 7. c | 9. j |
| 2. b | 4. f | 6. i | 8. a | 10. g |

5

IX. Medical Scramble

Unscramble the letters to form a medical term from the clues. Use the letters in squares to complete the bonus term. Answers are upside down at the bottom of the page.

1. Medical specialty treating pregnant women

___ ___ ☐ ___ ___ ___ ___ ___ ___ ☐   S T B S C O R I E T

2. Inflammation of the ear   ☐ ___ ___ ___ ___ ___   T I O S I T

3. Branch of medicine that uses operative methods

___ ___ ___ ___ ___ ___ ☐   G Y S R U E R

4. Pertaining to producing tumors

___ ___ ☐ ___ ___ ___ ___ ___ ___   C G N E O I N C O

5. Pertaining to treating children

☐ ___ ___ ___ ___ ___ ___ ☐ ___   T I E P R D C I A

6. Study of disease

___ ___ ___ ☐ ___ ___ ___ ___ ___   L A P G O H Y T O

7. New opening of the colon to the outside of the body

___ ___ ___ ___ ☐ ___ ___ ___ ___   O L M Y S O C O T

BONUS TERM: ABNORMAL CONDITION OF THE MIND

☐ ☐ ☐ ☐ ☐ ☐ ☐ ☐ ☐

Appendix

I

Body Systems

This appendix contains full-color diagrams of body systems. Each system contains six sections. **Anatomy** shows major organs and structures with labels and combining forms (in parenthesis) for each body part. The parts of the body are defined and explained in the *Glossary of Medical Terms* on p. 313. **Terminology** reviews combining forms and their meanings and gives examples of terminology using each combining form. **Pathology** explains terms related to common pathological conditions. **Laboratory Tests and Diagnostic Procedures** presents common tests and procedures, which can be cross-referenced for additional information in *Appendix II (Diagnostic Tests and Procedures)*. **Treatment Procedures** explains procedures that treat abnormal conditions in each system. **Matching Exercises and Answers** review the terminology to test your understanding.

Use this appendix as both a study guide for classroom work and as a reference for your work in the medical field.

I. CARDIOVASCULAR SYSTEM

Anatomy

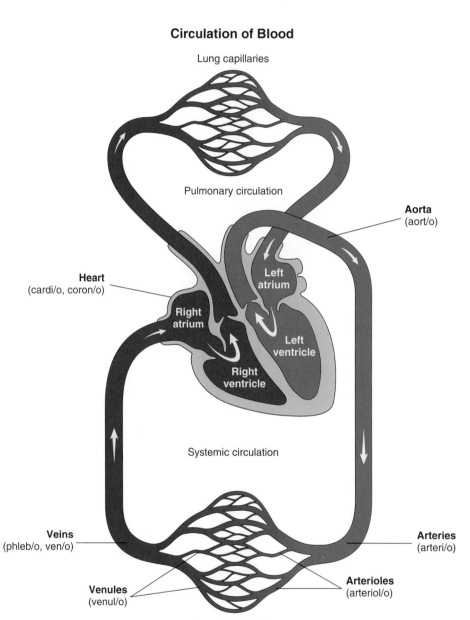

Circulation of Blood

Red vessels contain blood that is rich in oxygen. Arrows show the path of blood flow from the tissue capillaries through venules and veins toward the heart, to the lung capillaries, back to the heart, out the aorta to the arteries and arterioles, and then back to the tissue capillaries.

Terminology

Meanings for terminology are found in the *Glossary of Medical Terms*.

Combining Form	Meaning	Terminology	Meaning
angi/o	vessel	angioplasty	_____
aort/o	aorta	aortic stenosis	_____
arteri/o	artery	arteriosclerosis	_____
arteriol/o	arteriole	arteriolitis	_____
cardi/o	heart	cardiomyopathy	_____
coron/o	heart	coronary arteries	_____
phleb/o	vein	phlebotomy	_____
ven/o	vein	intravenous	_____
venul/o	venule	venulitis	_____

Pathology

Definitions for additional terms in boldface are found in the *Glossary of Medical Terms*.

Aneurysm: Local widening of an artery caused by weakness in the arterial wall or breakdown of the wall from **atherosclerosis.**

Angina: Chest pain caused by decreased blood flow to heart muscle. Also called angina pectoris (chest).

Arrhythmia: Abnormal heartbeat (rhythm); **fibrillation** and **flutter** are examples.

Atherosclerosis: Hardening of arteries with a collection of cholesterol-like plaque.

Congestive heart failure: Inability of the heart to pump its required amount of blood. Blood accumulates in the lungs, causing **pulmonary edema.**

Hypertension: High blood pressure. Essential hypertension is high blood pressure with no apparent cause. In secondary hypertension, another illness (kidney disease or an adrenal gland disorder) is the cause of the high blood pressure.

Myocardial infarction: Heart attack. An **infarction** is an area of dead **(necrotic)** tissue.

Shock: A group of symptoms (paleness of skin, weak and rapid pulse, shallow breathing) indicating poor oxygen supply to tissues and insufficient return of blood to the heart.

I. CARDIOVASCULAR SYSTEM (Continued)

Laboratory Tests and Diagnostic Procedures

Consult *Appendix II* for pronunciation of terms and additional information.

Angiography: Recording (via x-ray images) blood vessels after the injection of contrast into the bloodstream.

Cardiac catheterization: Introducing a catheter (a flexible, tubular instrument) into a vein or artery to measure pressure and flow patterns of blood.

Doppler ultrasound: Measuring blood flow in vessels via sound waves.

Echocardiography: Producing images of the heart via sound waves or echoes.

Electrocardiography: Recording electricity flowing through the heart.

Holter monitor: Detection of abnormal heart rhythms **(arrhythmias)** that involves having a patient wear a compact version of an electrocardiograph for 24 hours.

Lipid tests: Measurements of cholesterol and triglyceride levels in the blood.

Lipoprotein tests: Measurements of **high-density lipoprotein (HDL)** and **low-density lipoprotein (LDL)** in the blood.

Magnetic resonance imaging (MRI): Producing an image, by beaming magnetic waves at the heart, that gives detailed information about congenital heart disease, cardiac masses, and disease within large blood vessels.

MUGA scan: Imaging the motion of heart wall muscles and assessing the function of the heart via a *mu*ltiple-*g*ated *a*cquisition scan, which uses radioactive chemicals.

Positron emission tomography (PET scan): Radioactive chemicals, which release radioactive particles, are injected into the bloodstream and travel to the heart. Cross-sectional images show the flow of blood and the functional activity of the heart muscle.

Serum enzyme tests: Measurements of enzymes released into the bloodstream after a heart attack (myocardial infarction).

Stress test: An electrocardiogram plus blood pressure and heart rate measurements show the heart's response to physical exertion (treadmill test).

Technetium 99m Sestamibi scan: A radioactive chemical (technetium-99m Sestamibi) is injected intravenously and shows perfusion (flow) of blood in heart muscle. It is taken up in the area of a myocardial infarction, producing hot spots. In an ETT-MIBI (exercise tolerance test), IV radioactive substance is given before the patient reaches maximum heart rate on a treadmill.

Thallium-201 scan: A radioactive test that shows where thallium-201 (a radioactive substance) localizes in heart muscle.

Treatment Procedures

Cardioversion: Brief discharges of electricity passing across the chest to stop a cardiac **arrhythmia.** Also called **defibrillation.**

Coronary artery bypass graft (CABG):   Vessels taken from a patient's legs or chest are connected to coronary arteries to make detours around blockages.

Endarterectomy: Surgical removal of the innermost lining of an artery to remove fatty deposits and clots.

Heart transplantation: A donor heart is transferred to a recipient.

Percutaneous coronary intervention (PCI):   A balloon-tipped catheter (a flexible, tubular instrument) is threaded into a coronary artery to compress fatty deposits and open the artery. Stents (expandable slotted tubes) create wider openings that make the recurrence of blockages less likely. Also called **balloon angioplasty.**

Thrombolytic therapy: Drugs, such as tPA (tissue plasminogen activator) and streptokinase, are injected into a patient's bloodstream to dissolve clots that may cause a heart attack.

I. CARDIOVASCULAR SYSTEM (Continued)

Matching Exercises

The following exercises will help you review terminology related to the cardiovascular system. Answers are found on p. 274.

A. Match the term in Column I with its meaning in Column II.

Column I		Column II
1. aorta	_____	A. Blood vessels that carry blood to the heart from the body tissues
2. lung capillaries	_____	B. Largest artery in the body
3. arteries	_____	C. Tiny blood vessels that lie near cells and through whose walls gases, food, and wastes can pass
4. arterioles	_____	
5. venules	_____	D. Small veins
6. veins	_____	E. Small arteries
7. pulmonary circulation	_____	F. Blood vessels that carry blood away from the heart
8. systemic circulation	_____	G. Passage of blood from the heart to the body tissues and back
9. tissue capillaries	_____	H. Hollow muscular organ that pumps blood all over the body
10. heart	_____	I. Tiny blood vessels surrounding lung tissue through which gases pass into and out of the blood
		J. Passage of blood from the heart to the lungs and back to the heart

B. Match the combining form in Column I with its meaning in Column II.

Column I	Column II
1. phleb/o _____	A. Artery
2. arteriol/o _____	B. Vessel
3. angi/o _____	C. Heart
4. venul/o _____	D. Vein
5. arteri/o _____	E. Small artery
6. coron/o _____	F. Small vein

C. Match the medical term in Column I with its meaning in Column II.

Column I	Column II
1. intravenous _____	A. Inflammation of small veins
2. arteriosclerosis _____	B. Narrowing of the largest artery
3. phlebotomy _____	C. Disease of heart muscle
4. cardiomyopathy _____	D. Pertaining to within a vein
5. angioplasty _____	E. Inflammation of small arteries
6. arteriolitis _____	F. Hardening of arteries
7. venulitis _____	G. Incision of a vein
8. aortic stenosis _____	H. Surgical repair of blood vessels

I. CARDIOVASCULAR SYSTEM (Continued)

D. Match the pathological term in Column I with its meaning in Column II.

Column I	Column II
1. hypertension _____	A. Abnormal heartbeat
2. atherosclerosis _____	B. Local widening of an artery
3. angina _____	C. Heart attack
4. shock _____	D. Chest pain
5. myocardial infarction _____	E. High blood pressure
6. arrhythmia _____	F. Inability of the heart to pump its required amount of blood
7. congestive heart failure _____	G. Group of symptoms: pale skin, weak rapid pulse and shallow respirations
8. aneurysm _____	H. Hardening of arteries with cholesterol-like plaque

E. Match the test or procedure in Column I with its description in Column II.

Column I	Column II
1. lipid tests _____	A. Sound waves produce images of the heart
2. MUGA scan _____	B. X-ray images of blood vessels after contrast is injected into the bloodstream
3. lipoprotein tests _____	C. Measurement of HDL and LDL in blood
4. Holter monitor _____	
5. angiography _____	D. Recording electricity through the heart
6. serum enzyme tests _____	

7. electrocardiography ____

8. echocardiography ____

9. Sestamibi scan ____

10. Doppler ultrasound ____

E. Measurement of substances in the blood that indicate a heart attack

F. Sound waves measure blood flow in vessels

G. Abnormal heart rhythms are detected with a compact ECG over a 24-hour period

H. Radioactive test to detect blood perfusion in heart muscle

I. Measurement of triglyceride and cholesterol levels in the blood

J. Radioactive chemicals and a scanner produce images of the motion of the heart wall

F. Match the treatment procedure in Column I with its description in Column II.

Column I	Column II

1. cardioversion ____

2. thrombolytic therapy ____

3. heart transplantation ____

4. endarterectomy ____

5. CABG ____

6. PCI ____

A. Surgery to detour around blockages in coronary arteries

B. Drugs such as tPA dissolve clots that may cause a heart attack

C. Balloon-tipped catheter with stent opens coronary arteries

D. A donor heart is transferred to a recipient

E. Brief discharges of electricity stop a cardiac arrhythmia

F. Removal of innermost lining of an artery to eliminate fatty deposits

II. DIGESTIVE SYSTEM

Anatomy

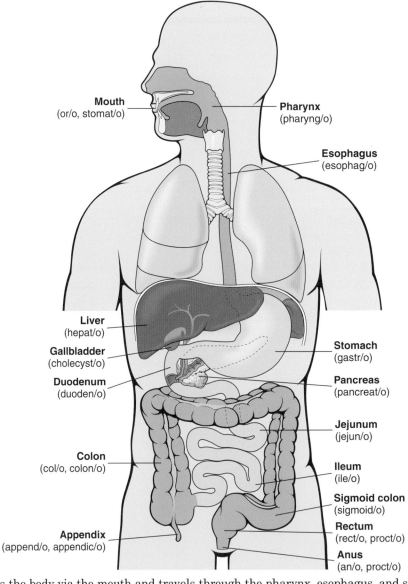

Mouth
(or/o, stomat/o)

Pharynx
(pharyng/o)

Esophagus
(esophag/o)

Liver
(hepat/o)

Gallbladder
(cholecyst/o)

Duodenum
(duoden/o)

Stomach
(gastr/o)

Pancreas
(pancreat/o)

Jejunum
(jejun/o)

Colon
(col/o, colon/o)

Ileum
(ile/o)

Sigmoid colon
(sigmoid/o)

Appendix
(append/o, appendic/o)

Rectum
(rect/o, proct/o)

Anus
(an/o, proct/o)

Food enters the body via the mouth and travels through the pharynx, esophagus, and stomach to the small intestine (duodenum). The liver, gallbladder, and pancreas make and store chemicals that aid in the digestion of foods. Digested (broken down) food is absorbed into the bloodstream through the walls of the small intestine (jejunum and ileum). Any food that cannot be absorbed continues into the colon (large intestine) and leaves the body through the rectum and anus. (Modified from Chabner D-E: *The Language of Medicine,* ed 7, Philadelphia, 2004, WB Saunders.)

Terminology

Meanings for terminology are found in the *Glossary of Medical Terms.*

Combining Form	Meaning	Terminology	Meaning
an/o	anus	anal _____	
append/o	appendix	appendectomy _____	
appendic/o	appendix	appendicitis _____	
cholecyst/o	gallbladder	cholecystectomy _____	
col/o	colon	colostomy _____	
colon/o	colon	colonoscopy _____	
duoden/o	duodenum	duodenal _____	
esophag/o	esophagus	esophageal _____	
gastr/o	stomach	gastralgia _____	
hepat/o	liver	hepatomegaly _____	
ile/o	ileum	ileostomy _____	
jejun/o	jejunum	gastrojejunostomy _____	
or/o	mouth	oral _____	
pancreat/o	pancreas	pancreatitis _____	
pharyng/o	pharynx	pharyngeal _____	
proct/o	anus and rectum	proctoscopy _____	
rect/o	rectum	rectocele _____	
sigmoid/o	sigmoid colon	sigmoidoscopy _____	
stomat/o	mouth	stomatitis _____	

II. DIGESTIVE SYSTEM (Continued)

Pathology

Definitions for additional terms in boldface are found in the *Glossary of Medical Terms*.

Cholelithiasis: Abnormal condition of gallstones.
Cirrhosis: Chronic disease of the liver with degeneration of liver cells.
Colonic polyposis: Condition in which **polyps** protrude from the mucous membrane lining the colon.
Diverticulosis: Abnormal condition of small pouches or sacs **(diverticula)** in the wall of the intestine (often the colon). **Diverticulitis** is inflammation and infection within diverticula.
Gastroesophageal reflux disease (GERD):   Backflow of the contents of the stomach into the esophagus.
Hepatitis: Inflammation of the liver.
Inflammatory bowel disease: Inflammation of the terminal (last) portion of the ileum **(Crohn disease)** or inflammation of the colon **(ulcerative colitis).**
Jaundice: Yellow-orange coloration of the skin and other tissues, from high levels of **bilirubin** in the bloodstream **(hyperbilirubinemia)**.

Laboratory Tests and Diagnostic Procedures

Consult *Appendix II* for pronunciation of terms and additional information.

Abdominal computed tomography (CT scan):   A series of cross-sectional x-ray images that show abdominal organs.
Abdominal magnetic resonance imaging (MRI):   Magnetic and radio waves create images of abdominal organs and tissues in all three planes of the body.
Abdominal ultrasound: Process of beaming sound waves into the abdomen to produce images of organs such as the gallbladder. **Endoscopic ultrasound** is useful to detect enlarged lymph nodes and tumors in the upper abdomen.
Barium tests: X-ray examinations using a liquid barium mixture to locate disorders of the gastrointestinal tract. In a **barium enema (lower GI series),** barium is injected into the anus and rectum and x-ray images are taken of the colon. In an **upper GI series (barium swallow),** barium is taken in through the mouth and x-ray images reveal the esophagus, stomach, and small intestine.
Cholangiography: X-ray examination of the bile ducts (CHOLANGI/O-) after the injection of contrast material through the liver **(percutaneous transhepatic cholangiography)** or through a catheter (a flexible, tubular instrument) from the mouth, esophagus, and stomach into the bile ducts **(endoscopic retrograde cholangiopancreatography or ERCP).**
Gastrointestinal endoscopy: Visual examination of the gastrointestinal tract with an endoscope. Examples are **esophagoscopy, gastroscopy,** and **sigmoidoscopy.**

Hemoccult test: Feces are placed on paper containing the chemical guaiac, which reacts with hidden (occult) blood. This is an important screening test for colon cancer.

Liver function tests (LFTs):   Measurements of liver enzymes and other substances in the blood. Enzyme levels increase when the liver is damaged (as in hepatitis). Examples of liver enzymes are **ALT (SGPT), AST (SGOT),** and **alkaline phosphatase (alk phos).** High **bilirubin** (blood pigment) levels indicate **jaundice** caused by liver disease or other problems affecting the liver.

Stool culture: Feces (stools) are placed in a growth medium (culture) to test for microorganisms (such as bacteria).

Treatment Procedures

Anastomosis: Surgical creation of an opening between two gastrointestinal organs. Examples are gastrojejunostomy, cholecystojejunostomy, and choledochoduodenostomy (CHOLEDOCH/O- means common bile duct).

Colostomy: Surgical creation of a new opening of the colon to the outside of the body.

Ileostomy: Surgical creation of a new opening of the ileum to the outside of the body.

Laparoscopic surgery: Removal of organs and tissues via a laparoscope (instrument inserted into the abdomen through a small incision). Examples are **laparoscopic cholecystectomy** and **laparoscopic appendectomy.** Also known as **minimally invasive surgery.**

II. DIGESTIVE SYSTEM (Continued)

Matching Exercises

The following exercises will help you review terminology related to the digestive system. Answers are found on pp. 274-275.

A. Match the term in Column I with its description in Column II.

Column I	Column II
1. mouth _____	A. Organ that receives food from the esophagus and sends it to the intestine
2. pharynx _____	B. Third part of the small intestine
3. esophagus _____	C. Throat
4. stomach _____	D. Second part of the small intestine
5. duodenum _____	E. Large intestine
6. jejunum _____	F. First part of the small intestine
7. ileum _____	G. Opening that is the beginning of the digestive system
8. colon _____	H. Tube that carries food to the stomach

B. Match the term in Column I with its description in Column II.

Column I	Column II
1. sigmoid colon _____	A. Opening of the colon to the outside of the body
2. rectum _____	B. Sac that stores bile
3. anus _____	C. S-shaped lower portion of the large intestine
4. appendix _____	D. Organ that makes bile, stores sugar, and produces proteins to clot blood
5. liver _____	

6. gallbladder _____

7. common bile duct _____

8. pancreas _____

E. Gland that makes both digestive juices and insulin (hormone)

F. Small sac that hangs from the beginning of the large intestine

G. Tube that carries bile from the liver and gallbladder to the intestine

H. Final section of the colon

C. Match the combining form in Column I with its meaning in Column II.

Column I	Column II
1. gastr/o _____	A. Mouth
2. col/o _____	B. Endocrine and exocrine gland near the stomach
3. proct/o _____	C. Third part of the small intestine
4. cholecyst/o _____	D. Stomach
5. pharyng/o _____	E. Liver
6. or/o _____	F. First part of the small intestine
7. hepat/o _____	G. Large intestine
8. duoden/o _____	H. Anus and rectum
9. ile/o _____	I. Gallbladder
10. pancreat/o _____	J. Throat

II. DIGESTIVE SYSTEM (Continued)

D. Match the term in Column I with its meaning in Column II.

Column I		Column II
1. hepatomegaly	_____	A. Pertaining to the tube leading from the throat to the stomach
2. cholecystectomy	_____	B. Pain of the stomach
3. proctoscopy	_____	
		C. Enlargement of the liver
4. ileostomy	_____	D. Inflammation of the mouth
5. stomatitis	_____	
		E. Pertaining to the first part of the small intestine
6. gastrojejunostomy	_____	
7. pancreatitis	_____	F. Removal of the gallbladder
8. duodenal	_____	G. Visual examination of the anus and rectum
9. esophageal	_____	H. New opening of the third part of the small intestine to the outside of the body
10. gastralgia	_____	
		I. New opening between the stomach and second part of the small intestine
		J. Inflammation of a gland adjacent to the stomach

E. Match the pathological term in Column I with its meaning in Column II.

Column I		Column II
1. hepatitis	_____	A. Yellow-orange coloration of the skin and other tissues
2. cirrhosis	_____	
		B. Abnormal condition of small pouches or sacs in the wall of the intestine
3. cholelithiasis	_____	
4. colonic polyposis	_____	C. Ulcerative colitis and Crohn disease

5. jaundice   _____

6. inflammatory bowel disease   _____

7. diverticulosis   _____

D. Inflammation of the liver

E. Abnormal condition of gallstones

F. Chronic disease of the liver with degeneration of liver cells

G. Small growths protrude from the mucous membrane lining the intestine

F. Match the test or procedure in Column I with its description in Column II.

Column I	Column II
1. LFTs _____	A. X-ray examination of bile ducts
2. abdominal CT _____	B. Minimally invasive surgery
3. cholangiography _____	C. Visual examination of the gastrointestinal tract (colonoscopy)
4. stool culture _____	D. Feces are placed in a growth medium and tested for microorganisms
5. GI endoscopy _____	E. Cholecystojejunostomy
6. stool guaiac _____	F. Magnetic waves create images of abdominal organs in three planes of the body
7. barium tests _____	G. Measurements of liver enzymes (ALT, AST, alk phos) and other substances
8. abdominal MRI _____	H. Feces are tested for blood
9. anastomosis _____	I. Series of cross-sectional x-ray images show abdominal organs
10. laparoscopic surgery _____	J. X-ray images of the GI tract after introducing a radiopaque liquid into the rectum or mouth

III. ENDOCRINE SYSTEM

Anatomy

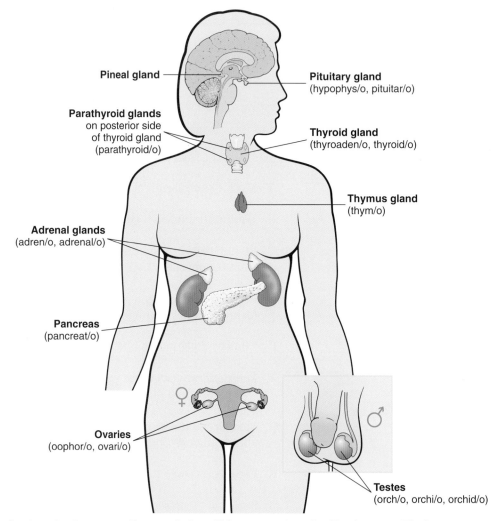

Endocrine glands secrete (form and give off) hormones into the bloodstream. The hormones travel throughout the body, affecting organs (including other endocrine glands) and controlling their actions. (Modified from Chabner D-E: *The Language of Medicine,* ed 7, Philadelphia, 2004, WB Saunders.)

Terminology

Meanings for terminology are found in the *Glossary of Medical Terms.*

Combining Form	Meaning	Terminology	Meaning
adren/o	adrenal gland	adrenopathy	_____
adrenal/o	adrenal gland	adrenalectomy	_____
hypophys/o	pituitary gland	hypophyseal	_____
oophor/o	ovary	oophoritis	_____
ovari/o	ovary	ovarian cyst	_____
orch/o	testis	orchitis	_____
orchi/o	testis	orchiopexy	_____
orchid/o	testis	orchidectomy	_____
pancreat/o	pancreas	pancreatectomy	_____
parathyroid/o	parathyroid gland	hyperparathyroidism	_____
pituitar/o	pituitary gland	hypopituitarism	_____
thym/o	thymus gland	thymoma	_____
thyroaden/o	thyroid gland	thyroadenitis	_____
thyroid/o	thyroid gland	thyroidectomy	_____

III. ENDOCRINE SYSTEM (Continued)

Pathology

Definitions for additional terms in boldface are found in the *Glossary of Medical Terms.*

Acromegaly: Enlargement of extremities caused by hypersecretion from the anterior portion of the pituitary gland after puberty.

Cushing syndrome: A group of symptoms produced by excess secretion of **cortisol** from the adrenal cortex. These symptoms include obesity, moon-like fullness of the face, **hyperglycemia,** and **osteoporosis.**

Diabetes mellitus: A disorder of the pancreas that causes an increase in blood glucose levels. **Type 1 diabetes,** with the onset usually in childhood, involves complete deficiency of **insulin** in the body. **Type 2 diabetes,** with the onset usually in adulthood, involves some insulin deficiency and resistance of tissues to the action of insulin.

Goiter: Enlargement of the thyroid gland.

Hyperthyroidism: Overactivity of the thyroid gland; also called **Graves disease** or **exophthalmic** (eyeballs bulge outward) **goiter.**

Laboratory Tests and Diagnostic Procedures

Consult *Appendix II* for pronunciation of terms and additional information.

Computed tomography (CT scan): Cross-sectional x-ray images of the pituitary gland and other endocrine organs.

Exophthalmometry: Measurement of eyeball protrusion **(exophthalmos)** as an indicator of **Graves disease (hyperthyroidism).**

Fasting blood sugar (glucose) test: Measurement of glucose levels in a blood sample taken from a fasting patient and in specimens taken 30 minutes, 1 hour, 2 hours, and 3 hours after the ingestion of 75 gm of glucose. Delayed return of blood glucose to normal levels indicates **diabetes mellitus.**

Magnetic resonance imaging (MRI): Magnetic waves produce images of the **hypothalamus,** pituitary gland, and other endocrine organs in all three planes of the body.

Radioactive iodine uptake: The uptake of radioactive iodine, given by mouth, measured as evidence of thyroid function.

Serum and urine tests: Measurement of hormones, **electrolytes,** and glucose levels in blood (serum) and urine as indicators of endocrine function.

Thyroid function tests: Measurement of levels of T_4 (thyroxine), T_3 (triiodothyronine), and TSH (thyroid-stimulating hormone) in the bloodstream.

Thyroid scan: Procedure in which a radioactive compound, injected intravenously, localizes in the thyroid gland. A scanning device produces an image showing the presence of tumors or nodules in the gland.

Matching Exercises

The following exercise will help you review terminology related to the endocrine system. Answers are found on p. 275.

A. Match the term in Column I with its location in Column II.

Column I		Column II
1. thyroid gland	*C*	A. Two paired male glands located in the scrotal sac
2. ovaries	*H*	
3. testes	*A*	B. Organ at the base of the brain in the sella turcica (round depression at the base of the skull)
4. thymus gland	*E*	
5. parathyroid glands	*G*	C. Gland in the neck on either side of the trachea
6. pituitary gland	*B*	
7. pancreas	*F*	D. Two glands, one above each kidney
8. adrenal glands	*D*	E. Gland in the middle of the chest (mediastinum)
		F. Gland adjacent to the stomach
		G. Four glands behind the thyroid gland
		H. Two paired organs in the female abdomen

III. ENDOCRINE SYSTEM (Continued)

B. **Match the combining form in Column I with the secretion or function in Column II.**

Column I		Column II
1. hypophys/o	F	A. Regulates calcium in the blood and bones
2. orchid/o	D	B. Secretes adrenaline and cortisone
3. thym/o	E	C. Secretes insulin, which allows sugar to enter cells
4. oophor/o	G	D. Secretes testosterone
5. thyroaden/o	H	E. Secretes thymosin and produces white blood cells
6. pancreat/o	C	F. Secretes growth hormone and hormones that control the thyroid gland, ovaries, and testes
7. adren/o	B	G. Secretes estrogen and progesterone
8. parathyroid/o	A	H. Secretes thyroxine (T_4), which increases metabolism of body cells

C. **Match the medical term in Column I with its meaning in Column II.**

Column I		Column II
1. thyroadenitis	D	A. Disease of the adrenal glands
2. oophoritis	H	B. Tumor of the thymus gland
3. orchiopexy	F	C. Pertaining to the pituitary gland
4. thymoma	B	D. Inflammation of the thyroid gland
5. hyperparathyroidism	G	E. Removal of the thyroid gland
6. thyroidectomy	E	F. Surgical fixation of an undescended testicle
7. adrenopathy	A	G. Increased secretion of parathyroid hormone
8. hypophyseal	C	H. Inflammation of an ovary

D. Match the pathological condition in Column I with its description in Column II.

Column I	Column II
1. diabetes mellitus _C_	A. Enlargement of the thyroid gland
2. acromegaly _D_	B. Hypersecretion of cortisone from the adrenal glands
3. goiter _A_	C. Deficiency of insulin leading to high blood sugar levels
4. Cushing syndrome _B_	D. Enlargement of extremities caused by increased growth hormone from the pituitary gland
5. hyperthyroidism _E_	E. Overactivity of the thyroid gland

E. Match the test or procedure in Column I with its description in Column II.

Column I	Column II
1. thyroid scan _B_	A. Measures blood glucose levels
2. exophthalmometry _E_	B. Radioactive compound, injected intravenously, localizes in the thyroid gland; images are produced
3. fasting blood sugar _A_	
4. thyroid function tests _G_	C. Measures hormones, electrolytes, and sugar in blood and urine
5. CT scan _F_	D. Measures localization of an element necessary for making thyroid hormone
6. serum and urine tests _C_	E. Measures eyeball protrusion
7. radioactive iodine uptake _D_	F. Cross-sectional x-rays of endocrine organs
	G. Measures T_3, T_4, and TSH levels in the blood

IV. FEMALE REPRODUCTIVE SYSTEM

Anatomy

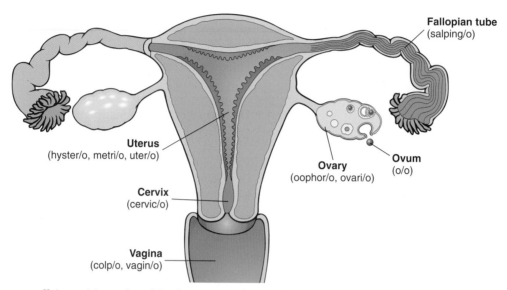

Fallopian tube
(salping/o)

Uterus
(hyster/o, metri/o, uter/o)

Ovary
(oophor/o, ovari/o)

Ovum
(o/o)

Cervix
(cervic/o)

Vagina
(colp/o, vagin/o)

An egg cell (ovum) is produced in the ovary and travels through the fallopian tube. If a sperm cell is present and fertilization (the union of the egg and sperm cell) takes place, the resulting cell (embryo) may implant in the lining of the uterus. The embryo (later called the fetus) develops in the uterus for nine months and is delivered from the body through the cervix and vagina. (Modified from Chabner D-E: *The Language of Medicine,* ed 7, Philadelphia, 2004, WB Saunders.)

Terminology

Meanings for terminology are found in the *Glossary of Medical Terms*.

Combining Form	Meaning	Terminology	Meaning
cervic/o	cervix	cervical _____	
colp/o	vagina	colposcopy _____	
vagin/o	vagina	vaginitis _____	
hyster/o	uterus	hysterectomy _____	
metri/o	uterus	endometrium _____	
uter/o	uterus	uterine _____	
o/o	egg	oocyte _____	
oophor/o	ovary	oophorectomy _____	
ovari/o	ovary	ovarian cancer _____	
salping/o	fallopian tube	salpingectomy _____	

Pathology

Definitions for additional terms in boldface are found in the *Glossary of Medical Terms*.

Amenorrhea: Absence of menstrual flow.

Dysmenorrhea: Painful menstrual flow.

Ectopic pregnancy: Pregnancy that is not in the uterus; usually occurring in a fallopian tube.

Endometriosis: Tissue from the inner lining of the uterus (**endometrium**) occurs abnormally in other pelvic or abdominal locations (**fallopian tubes, ovaries,** or **peritoneum**).

Fibroids: Benign tumors in the uterus. Also called a **leiomyoma;** LEI/O means smooth (referring to a **visceral muscle** within an internal organ).

Menorrhagia: Excessive discharge (-RRHAGIA) of blood from the uterus during **menstruation.**

Pelvic inflammatory disease: Inflammation (often caused by bacterial infection) in the region of the pelvis. Because the condition primarily affects the fallopian tubes, it is also called **salpingitis.**

IV. FEMALE REPRODUCTIVE SYSTEM (Continued)

Laboratory Tests and Diagnostic Procedures

Consult *Appendix II* for pronunciation of terms and additional information.

Amniocentesis: Surgical puncture of the amniotic sac (surrounding the fetus) to withdraw fluid for chemical and chromosomal analysis.

Aspiration: Withdrawal of fluid from a cavity or sac. In breast aspiration, a needle is used to remove fluid from cystic lesions in the breast. The fluid is analyzed for the presence of malignant cells.

Colposcopy: Visual examination of the vagina and cervix with a colposcope (a small, magnifying instrument resembling a mounted pair of binoculars).

Conization: Removal of a cone-shaped section of the cervix for **biopsy.**

Hysterosalpingography: X-ray imaging of the uterus and fallopian tubes after injection of a contrast material into the uterus.

Mammography: X-ray imaging of the breast.

Pap smear: Procedure in which a physician inserts a wooden spatula or cotton swab to take secretions from the cervix and vagina. Microscopic analysis of the smear (spread on a glass slide) indicates the presence of cervical or vaginal disease.

Pelvic ultrasonography: Procedure that produces an image of sound waves as they bounce off organs (such as the ovaries and uterus) in the pelvic (hip) region. In **transvaginal ultrasound,** a sound probe is placed in the vagina.

Pregnancy test: Measurement of human chorionic gonadotropin (HCG), a hormone in blood and urine that indicates pregnancy.

Treatment Procedures

Cauterization: The use of heat to destroy abnormal tissue, such as can occur, for example, in the lining of the **cervix** (lower neck-like region of the uterus).

Cryosurgery: The use of cold temperatures (liquid nitrogen) to freeze and destroy tissue (such as the lining of the cervix).

Dilation and curettage (D&C): Widening (dilation) of the opening of the cervix and scraping (curettage) of the lining of the uterus to remove tissue and stop prolonged or heavy uterine bleeding.

Myomectomy: The removal of **fibroid (myoma)** tissue from the uterus.

Tubal ligation: Procedure in which both fallopian tubes are ligated (tied off) in two places with sutures and the intervening segment is burned or removed. This prevents pregnancy.

Matching Exercises

The following exercises will help you review terminology related to the female reproductive system. Answers are found on pp. 275-276.

A. Match the term in Column I with its meaning in Column II.

Column I	Column II
1. ovary _____	A. Muscular passageway from the uterus to the outside of the body
2. cervix _____	B. Neck (lower portion) of the uterus
3. fallopian tube _____	C. One of two paired organs in the female abdomen that produces egg cells and hormones
4. vagina _____	D. One of two paired tubes that lead from the ovaries to the uterus
5. uterus _____	E. One of two paired glands in the front of the chest that produces milk after childbirth
6. breast _____	F. Muscular organ that holds and provides nourishment for the developing fetus

B. Match the combining form in Column I with its meaning in Column II.

Column I	Column II
1. oophor/o _____	A. Uterus
2. colp/o _____	B. Fallopian tube
3. salping/o _____	C. Neck of the uterus
4. hyster/o _____	D. Ovary
5. cervic/o _____	E. Vagina
6. mast/o _____	F. Breast

IV. FEMALE REPRODUCTIVE SYSTEM (Continued)

C. Match the medical term in Column I with its meaning in Column II.

Column I		Column II
1. salpingectomy	_____	A. Visual examination of the vagina
2. mammography	_____	B. Pertaining to the lower, neck-like region of the uterus
3. vaginitis	_____	
4. colposcopy	_____	C. Inflammation of the breast
		D. Removal of a fallopian tube
5. hysterectomy	_____	
6. cervical	_____	E. Inner lining of the uterus
7. endometrium	_____	F. X-ray imaging of the breast
		G. Resection of the uterus
8. mastitis	_____	
		H. Inflammation of the vagina

D. Match the pathological term in Column I with its meaning in Column II.

Column I		Column II
1. fibroids	_____	A. Absence of menstrual flow
2. dysmenorrhea	_____	B. Excessive discharge of blood from the uterus between menstrual periods
3. endometriosis	_____	
4. ectopic pregnancy	_____	C. Leiomyomas (benign muscle growths) in the uterus
5. amenorrhea	_____	D. Uterine tissue found in sites (ovary, fallopian tubes) other than in the uterus
6. pelvic inflammatory disease	_____	
		E. Painful menstrual flow
7. menorrhagia	_____	F. Salpingitis
		G. Embryo develops outside the uterus

E. Match the test or procedure in Column I with its description in Column II.

Column I		Column II
1. pregnancy test	_____	A. Endoscopic visual examination of the vagina
2. pelvic ultrasonography	_____	B. Withdrawal of fluid from a cavity or sac
3. conization	_____	C. Removal of a section of the cervix for biopsy
4. colposcopy	_____	D. X-ray imaging of the breast
5. mammography	_____	E. X-ray examination of the uterus and fallopian tubes
6. Pap smear	_____	
7. hysterosalpingography	_____	F. Sound wave image of organs in the hip region
8. aspiration	_____	G. Secretions from the vagina and cervix are examined microscopically
9. amniocentesis	_____	H. Measurement of HCG levels
		I. Surgical puncture to remove fluid from the sac surrounding the fetus

F. Match the treatment procedure in Column I with its description in Column II.

Column I		Column II
1. myomectomy	_____	A. Use of cold temperatures to freeze and destroy tissue
2. cryosurgery	_____	B. Fallopian tubes are tied to prevent pregnancy
3. cauterization	_____	C. Removal of fibroids from the uterus
4. tubal ligation	_____	D. Widening the cervix and scraping the lining of the uterus
5. D&C	_____	E. Use of heat to destroy abnormal tissue

V. LYMPHATIC SYSTEM

Anatomy

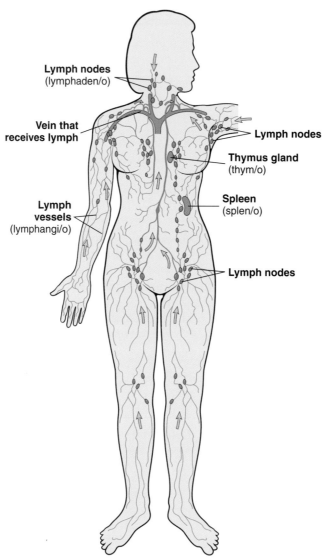

Lymph nodes
(lymphaden/o)

**Vein that
receives lymph**

**Lymph
vessels**
(lymphangi/o)

Lymph nodes

Thymus gland
(thym/o)

Spleen
(splen/o)

Lymph nodes

Lymph originates in the tissue spaces around cells and travels in lymph vessels and through lymph nodes to a large vein in the neck, where it enters the bloodstream. Lymph contains white blood cells (lymphocytes) that help the body fight disease. The spleen produces lymphocytes and disposes of dying blood cells. The thymus gland also produces lymphocytes. (Modified from Chabner D-E: *The Language of Medicine,* ed 7, Philadelphia, 2004, WB Saunders.)

Terminology

Meanings for terminology are found in the *Glossary of Medical Terms.*

Combining Form	Meaning	Terminology	Meaning
lymph/o	lymph fluid	lymphoma	_____
lymphaden/o	lymph node ("gland")	lymphadenectomy	_____
		lymphadenopathy	_____
lymphangi/o	lymph vessel	lymphangiectasis	_____
splen/o	spleen	splenomegaly	_____
thym/o	thymus gland	thymoma	_____

Pathology

Definitions for additional terms in boldface are found in the *Glossary of Medical Terms.*

Acquired immunodeficiency syndrome (AIDS): Suppression or deficiency of the immune response (destruction of **lymphocytes**) caused by exposure to **human immunodeficiency virus (HIV).**

Lymphoma: Malignant tumor of lymph nodes and lymphatic tissue. **Hodgkin disease** is an example of a lymphoma.

Mononucleosis: Acute infectious disease with enlargement of lymph nodes and increased numbers of **lymphocytes** and **monocytes** in the bloodstream.

Sarcoidosis: Inflammatory disease in which small nodules, or tubercles, form in lymph nodes and other organs. SARC/O- means flesh, and -OID means resembling.

Laboratory Tests and Diagnostic Procedures

Consult *Appendix II* for pronunciation of terms and additional information.

Computed tomography (CT scan): X-ray views in the transverse plane for the diagnosis of abnormalities in lymphoid organs (lymph nodes, spleen, and thymus gland).

ELISA (enzyme-*l*inked *i*mmuno*s*orbent *a*ssay): A test to screen for antibodies to the **human immunodeficiency virus,** which causes **acquired immunodeficiency syndrome (AIDS).**

Western blot test: A blood test to detect the presence of antibodies to specific antigens such as the **human immunodeficiency virus (HIV).** It is regarded as a more precise test than the ELISA.

V. LYMPHATIC SYSTEM (Continued)

Treatment Procedures

Chemotherapy: Treatment with powerful drugs to kill cancer cells (**Hodgkin disease, non-Hodgkin lymphoma,** and **multiple myeloma**) and viruses such as the **human immunodeficiency virus.**

Radiotherapy (radiation therapy):   Treatment with high-dose radiation to destroy malignant lesions in the body.

Matching Exercises

The following exercises will help you review terminology related to the lymphatic system. Answers are found on p. 276.

A. Match the term in Column I with its meaning in Column II.

Column I		Column II
1. lymph nodes	_____	A. Blood-forming organ in early life; later a storage organ for red blood cells and a source of lymphocytes
2. thymus	_____	
3. lymph	_____	B. Gland in the mediastinum; produces lymphocytes that play an important role in immunity
4. spleen	_____	
5. lymph vessels	_____	C. Stationary collections of lymph tissue throughout the body
		D. Clear fluid that bathes tissue spaces and circulates in lymph vessels
		E. Small tubes that carry lymph fluid throughout the body

B. Match the combining form in Column I with its meaning in Column II.

Column I		Column II
1. thym/o	_____	A. Spleen
2. lymphangi/o	_____	B. Lymph fluid
3. lymphaden/o	_____	C. Thymus gland

4. splen/o _____

5. lymph/o _____

D. Lymph vessels

E. Lymph nodes (glands)

C. Match the medical term in Column I with its meaning in Column II.

Column I	Column II
1. lymphadenopathy _____	A. Malignant tumor of lymph nodes and lymphatic tissue
2. lymphangiectasis _____	
3. splenomegaly _____	B. Acute infectious disease with enlargement of lymph nodes and increase in lymphocytes and monocytes
4. lymphoma _____	C. Malignant tumor of a mediastinal lymphocyte-producing gland
5. lymphadenectomy _____	
6. mononucleosis _____	D. Widening, dilation of lymph vessels
7. thymoma _____	E. Enlargement of an abdominal organ that produces lymphocytes
	F. Excision of lymph nodes
	G. Disease of lymph nodes

D. Match the procedure or test in Column I with its description in Column II.

Column I	Column II
1. ELISA _____	A. Treatment with high-dose radiation to destroy malignant tissue
2. Western blot _____	
3. chemotherapy _____	B. X-ray images in a cross-sectional plane for diagnosis of lymph node abnormalities
4. CT scan _____	C. Precise blood test to detect antibodies to specific antigens as in HIV
5. radiotherapy _____	
	D. Screening test for antibodies to the AIDS virus
	E. Treatment with powerful drugs to kill cancer cells

VI. MALE REPRODUCTIVE SYSTEM

Anatomy

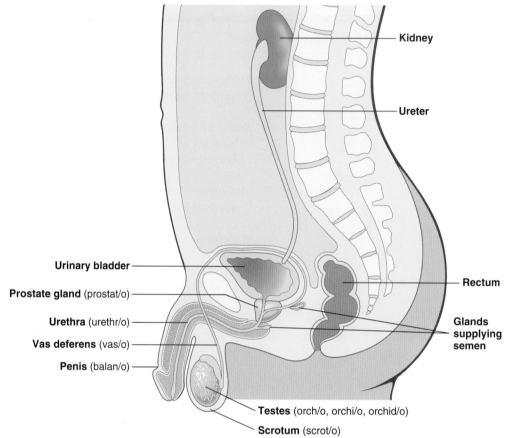

Sperm cells are produced in the testes (singular: testis) and travel up into the body, through the vas deferens, and around the urinary bladder. The vas deferens unites with the urethra, which opens to the outside of the body through the penis. The prostate and the other glands near the urethra produce a fluid (semen) that leaves the body with sperm cells. (Modified from Chabner D-E: *The Language of Medicine,* ed 7, Philadelphia, 2004, WB Saunders.)

Terminology

Meanings for terminology are found in the *Glossary of Medical Terms*.

Combining Form	Meaning	Terminology	Meaning
balan/o	penis	balanitis _____	
orch/o	testis	orchitis _____	
orchi/o	testis	orchiectomy _____	
orchid/o	testis	orchidectomy _____	
prostat/o	prostate gland	prostatectomy _____	
scrot/o	scrotum	scrotal _____	
urethr/o	urethra	urethritis _____	
vas/o	vas deferens	vasectomy _____	

Pathology

Definitions for additional terms in boldface are found in the *Glossary of Medical Terms*.

Benign prostatic hyperplasia: Noncancerous enlargement of the prostate gland. Also called **benign prostatic hypertrophy.**

Cryptorchism: Condition of undescended testis. The testis is not in the scrotal sac at birth. CRYPT/O- means hidden.

Hydrocele: Sac of clear fluid in the scrotum. HYDR/O- means water, and -CELE indicates a hernia (a bulging or swelling).

Prostatic carcinoma: Cancer of the prostate gland (prostate cancer).

Testicular carcinoma: Malignant tumor of the testis. An example is a **seminoma.**

Varicocele: Enlarged, swollen veins near a testicle. VARIC/O- means swollen veins.

VI. MALE REPRODUCTIVE SYSTEM (Continued)

Laboratory Tests and Diagnostic Procedures

Consult *Appendix II* for pronunciation of terms and additional information.

Digital rectal examination (DRE):   Examination of the prostate gland with finger palpation through the rectum.

Prostate-specific antigen (PSA):   Measurement of the amount of PSA in the blood. Higher than normal levels are associated with prostatic enlargement and prostate cancer.

Semen analysis: Measurement of the number, shape, and motility (ability to move) of sperm cells.

Treatment Procedures

Orchiopexy: Surgical fixation (-PEXY) of an undescended testicle in a young male infant.

Transurethral resection of the prostate gland (TURP):   The removal of portions of the prostate gland with an **endoscope** inserted into the urethra.

Vasectomy: Procedure in which the vas deferens on each side is cut, a piece is removed, and the free ends are folded and ligated (tied) with sutures. Vasectomy produces sterilization so that sperm are not released with semen.

Matching Exercises

The following exercises will help you review terminology related to the male reproductive system. Answers are found on pp. 276-277.

A. Match the term in Column I with its meaning in Column II.

Column I	Column II
1. scrotum _____	A. One of two paired male organs in the scrotum that produces sperm cells and male hormones
2. penis _____	B. External male organ, containing the urethra, through which both urine and semen (sperm cells and fluid) leave the body
3. vas deferens _____	
4. testis _____	C. Sac on the outside of the body that contains the testes
5. prostate _____	D. One of two tubes that carry sperm cells from the testes to the outside of the body
	E. Male organ that surrounds the base of the urinary bladder and produces fluid that leaves the body with sperm

B. Match the combining form in Column I with its meaning in Column II.

Column I	Column II
1. prostat/o _____	A. Tube leading from the urinary bladder to the outside of the body
2. vas/o _____	B. Gland that produces fluid portion of semen
3. orch/o _____	C. Penis
4. scrot/o _____	D. Testis
5. balan/o _____	E. Tube carrying sperm cells from the testis to the ejaculatory duct and urethra
6. urethra/o _____	F. Sac containing the testes

VI. MALE REPRODUCTIVE SYSTEM (Continued)

C. Match the medical term in Column I with its meaning in Column II

Column I		Column II
1. urethritis	_____	A. Resection of the prostate gland
2. scrotal	_____	B. Inflammation of the penis
3. vasectomy	_____	C. Inflammation of a testis
4. orchitis	_____	D. Inflammation of the urethra
5. prostatectomy	_____	E. Pertaining to the sac containing the testes
6. orchidectomy	_____	F. Resection of pieces of each vas deferens
7. balanitis	_____	G. Excision of a testicle

D. Match the pathological term in Column I with its meaning in Column II.

Column I		Column II
1. varicocele	_____	A. Undescended testicle
2. benign prostate hyperplasia	_____	B. Malignant tumor of the prostate gland
3. hydrocele	_____	C. Hernia (collection of fluid) in the scrotal sac
4. testicular carcinoma	_____	D. Malignant tumor; one type is a seminoma
5. prostatic carcinoma	_____	E. Swollen, twisted veins near the testis
6. cryptorchism	_____	F. Nonmalignant enlargement of the prostate gland

E. Match the test or procedure in Column I with its description in Column II.

Column I	Column II
1. orchiopexy _____	A. Measurement of the number, shape, and motility of sperm cells
2. vasectomy _____	B. Measures blood levels of prostate-specific antigen
3. TURP _____	C. Examination of the prostate gland with finger palpation through the rectum
4. DRE _____	D. Removal of portions of the prostate gland with an endoscope inserted into the urethra
5. semen analysis _____	E. Surgical fixation of an undescended testicle
6. PSA test _____	F. Two tubes that carry sperm from the testicles are cut and tied off

VII. MUSCULOSKELETAL SYSTEM

Anatomy

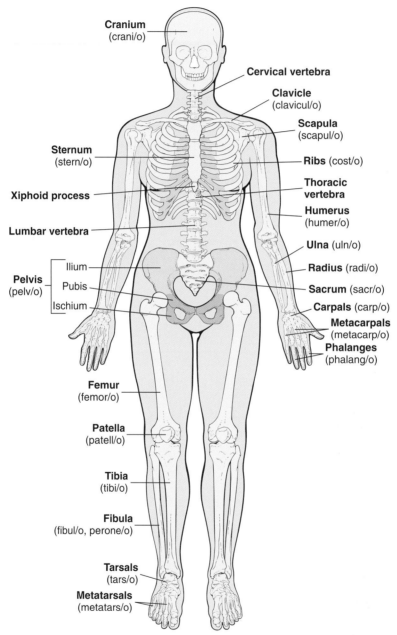

Bones are connected to muscles that contract to move the body. Joints are the spaces between bones. Near the joints are ligaments that connect bones to other bones and tendons that connect bones to muscles. (Modified from Chabner D-E: *The Language of Medicine,* ed 7, Philadelphia, 2004, WB Saunders.)

For your reference, included here are anterior and posterior views of superficial muscles in the body.

The anterior superficial muscles. (Modified from Miller-Keane: *Encyclopedia and Dictionary of Medicine, Nursing, and Allied Health,* ed 7, Philadelphia, 2003, WB Saunders.)

VII. MUSCULOSKELETAL SYSTEM (Continued)

Orbicularis oculi

Sternocleidomastoid

Masseter

Buccinator

Trapezius

Deltoid

Triceps brachii

Brachioradialis

Biceps brachii

Brachialis

Rhomboideus major

Latissimus dorsi

External oblique

Gluteus maximus

Adductor magnus

Gracilis

Biceps femoris

Gastrocnemius

Soleus

Achilles tendon

The posterior superficial muscles. (Modified from Miller-Keane: *Encyclopedia and Dictionary of Medicine, Nursing, and Allied Health,* ed 7, Philadelphia, 2003, WB Saunders.)

Terminology

Meanings for terminology are found in the *Glossary of Medical Terms*.

Combining Form	Meaning	Terminology	Meaning
arthr/o	joint	arthroscopy	_____
chondr/o	cartilage	chondroma	_____
cost/o	rib	costochondritis	_____
crani/o	skull	craniotomy	_____
ligament/o	ligament	ligamentous	_____
my/o	muscle	myosarcoma	_____
myos/o	muscle	myositis	_____
muscul/o	muscle	muscular	_____
myel/o	bone marrow	myelodysplasia	_____
oste/o	bone	osteomyelitis	_____
pelv/o	pelvis, hipbone	pelvic	_____
spondyl/o	vertebra	spondylosis	_____
vertebr/o	vertebra	intervertebral	_____
ten/o	tendon	tenorrhaphy	_____
tendin/o	tendon	tendinitis	_____

VII. MUSCULOSKELETAL SYSTEM (Continued)

Pathology

Definitions for additional terms in boldface are found in the *Glossary of Medical Terms.*

Ankylosing spondylitis: Chronic, progressive **arthritis** with stiffening **(ankylosis)** of joints, primarily of the spine and hip.

Carpal tunnel syndrome: Compression of the median nerve as it passes between the ligament and the bones and tendons of the wrist.

Gouty arthritis: Inflammation of joints caused by excessive uric acid. Also called **gout.**

Muscular dystrophy: An inherited disorder characterized by progressive weakness and degeneration of muscle fibers.

Osteoporosis: Decrease in bone density with thinning and weakening of bone. -POROSIS means containing passages or spaces.

Rheumatoid arthritis: Chronic inflammation of joints; pain, swelling, and stiffening, especially in the small joints of the hands and feet. RHEUMAT/O means flowing, descriptive of the swelling in joints.

Laboratory Tests and Diagnostic Procedures

Consult *Appendix II* for pronunciation of terms and additional information.

Antinuclear antibody test (ANA): Test in which a sample of plasma is tested for the presence of antibodies found in patients with systemic lupus erythematosus.

Arthrocentesis: Surgical puncture to remove fluid from a joint.

Arthrography: X-ray imaging of a joint.

Arthroscopy: Visual examination of a joint with an arthroscope.

Bone density test: Low-energy x-rays are taken of bones in the spinal column, pelvis, and wrist to detect areas of bone deficiency.

Bone scan: Procedure in which a radioactive substance is injected intravenously and its uptake in bones is measured with a special scanning device.

Calcium: Measurement of the amount of calcium in a sample of blood (serum). This test is important in evaluating diseases of bone.

Electromyography (EMG): Recording of the strength of muscle contraction as a result of electrical stimulation.

Erythrocyte sedimentation rate (ESR): Measurement of the rate at which red blood cells fall to the bottom of a test tube. High sedimentation rates are associated with inflammatory diseases such as **rheumatoid arthritis.**

Muscle biopsy: The removal of muscle tissue for microscopic examination.

Uric acid test: Measurement of the amount of uric acid in a sample of blood. High uric acid levels are associated with gouty arthritis.

Treatment Procedures

Arthroplasty: Surgical repair of a joint. Total hip arthroplasty is the replacement of the head of the femur (thigh bone) and acetabulum (cup-shaped portion of the hip socket) with artificial parts **(prostheses)** that are cemented into the bone.

Chemonucleolysis: Treatment of a herniated disk by injection of chymopapain to dissolve the inner portion (nucleus) of the disk.

Endoscopic diskectomy: Surgical removal of a herniated intervertebral disk with an endoscope.

Laminectomy: Surgical removal of a portion of a vertebra to allow visualization and removal of a portion of a protruding disk.

Microscopic diskectomy: Surgical removal of a herniated intervertebral disk with an incision that is 1 to 2 inches long and visualization of the surgical field with an operating microscope.

VII. MUSCULOSKELETAL SYSTEM (Continued)

Matching Exercises

The following exercises will help you review terminology related to the musculoskeletal system. Answers are found on p. 277.

A. Match the term in Column I with its description in Column II.

Column I		Column II
1. cranium	H	A. Finger bones
2. clavicle	E	B. Thigh bone
3. humerus	K	C. Kneecap
4. radius	D	D. Lower arm bone on the thumb side
5. ulna	J	E. Collar bone
6. carpals	R	F. Tailbone
7. metacarpals	Q	G. Breast bone
8. phalanges	A	H. Skull bone
9. scapula	T	I. Ankle bones
10. sternum	G	J. Lower arm bone (little finger side)
11. tarsals	I	K. Upper arm bone
12. metatarsals	S	L. Smaller of the lower leg bones
13. fibula	L	M. Hipbone
14. tibia	P	N. Lower part of the backbone near the hip
15. patella	C	O. Bones surrounding the chest cavity
16. sacrum	N	P. Larger of the lower leg bones

17. coccyx   _F_   Q. Hand bones

18. pelvis   _M_   R. Wrist bones

19. femur   _B_   S. Foot bones

20. ribs   _O_   T. Shoulder bone

B. Match the combining form in Column I with its meaning in Column II.

Column I		Column II
1. crani/o	_D_	A. Backbone
2. arthr/o	_C_	B. Cartilage
3. oste/o	_H_	C. Joint
4. cost/o	_E_	D. Skull
5. pelv/o	_G_	E. Rib
6. my/o	_F_	F. Muscle
7. ten/o	_I_	G. Hipbone
8. chondr/o	_B_	H. Bone
9. spondyl/o	_A_	I. Connects muscles to bones
10. ligament/o	_J_	J. Connects bones to other bones

VII. MUSCULOSKELETAL SYSTEM (Continued)

C. Match the medical term in Column I with its meaning in Column II.

Column I		Column II
1. myelodysplasia	G	A. Incision of the skull
2. intervertebral	E	B. Inflammation of cartilage attached to ribs
3. osteomyelitis	D	C. Suture of a tendon
4. arthroscopy	I	D. Inflammation of bone and bone marrow
5. costochondritis	B	E. Pertaining to between the backbones
6. chondroma	F	F. Benign tumor of cartilage tissue
7. tenorrhaphy	C	G. Abnormal growth of bone marrow cells
8. myosarcoma	H	H. Malignant tumor of muscle tissue
9. craniotomy	A	I. Visual examination of a joint

D. Match the pathological term in Column I with its meaning in Column II.

Column I	Column II
1. gouty arthritis _C_	A. Chronic, progressive arthritis with stiffening of joints between the backbones
2. carpal tunnel syndrome _B_	B. Compression of the median nerve in the wrist
3. rheumatoid arthritis _E_	C. High levels of uric acid with inflammation of joints
4. osteoporosis _F_	D. Weakness and degeneration of muscle fibers; congenital condition
5. ankylosing spondylitis _A_	E. Chronic inflammation of joints, especially small bones in the hands and feet
6. muscular dystrophy _D_	F. Decrease in bone density with thinning and weakening of bone

VII. MUSCULOSKELETAL SYSTEM (Continued)

E. Match the test or procedure in Column I with its description in Column II.

Column I		Column II
1. arthrocentesis	*E*	A. Recording the strength of muscle contraction
2. serum calcium	*G*	
3. electromyography	*A*	B. Measures sedimentation rate of red blood cells; indicates inflammation
4. bone scan	*F*	C. Plasma is tested for antibodies that are present in patients with systemic lupus erythematosus
5. ESR	*B*	
6. ANA test	*C*	D. Removal of muscle tissue for microscopic analysis
7. muscle biopsy	*D*	E. Surgical puncture to remove fluid from a joint
8. uric acid test	*I*	
9. arthroscopy	*J*	F. Radioactive substance is injected intravenously and uptake is measured in bone tissue
10. arthrography	*H*	

G. Measurement of an element in the blood that is necessary for normal bone formation

H. X-ray imaging of a joint

I. Measurement of the amount of a substance in blood that is associated with gouty arthritis

J. Visual examination of a joint using an endoscope

F. **Match the treatment procedure in Column I with its description in Column II.**

Column I		Column II
1. laminectomy	_D_	A. Surgical repair of a joint
2. microscopic diskectomy	_C_	B. Treatment of a herniated disk with a chemical to dissolve the inner portion of the disk
3. arthroplasty	_A_	
4. chemonucleolysis	_B_	C. Removal of a herniated disk using a tiny incision and an operating microscope
5. endoscopic diskectomy	_E_	

D. Surgical removal of a portion of a vertebra to allow visualization and removal of a portion of a disk

E. Surgical removal of a herniated disk with an endoscope

VIII. NERVOUS SYSTEM

Anatomy

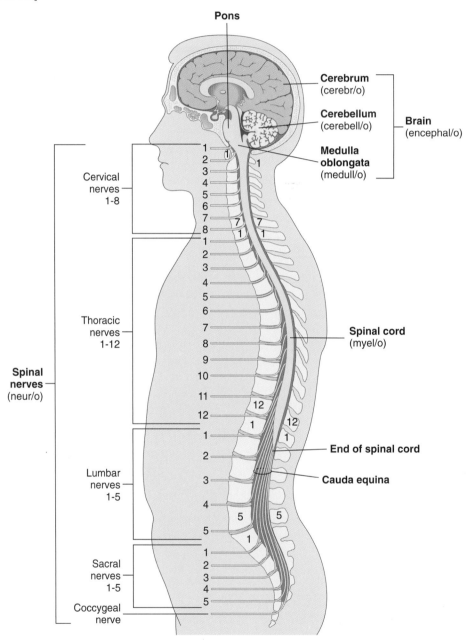

The central nervous system consists of the brain and the spinal cord. The peripheral nervous system includes the nerves that carry messages to and from the brain and spinal cord. Spinal nerves carry messages to and from the spinal cord, and the cranial nerves (not pictured) carry messages to and from the brain.

Terminology

Meanings for terminology are found in the *Glossary of Medical Terms*.

Combining Form	Meaning	Terminology	Meaning
cerebell/o	cerebellum	cerebellar	_____
cerebr/o	cerebrum	cerebral	_____
encephal/o	brain	encephalitis	_____
medull/o	medulla oblongata	medullary	_____
myel/o	spinal cord	myelitis	_____
neur/o	nerve	neuropathy	_____

Pathology

Definitions for additional terms in boldface are found in the *Glossary of Medical Terms*.

Alzheimer disease: Brain disorder marked by deterioration of mental capacity **(dementia).**

Cerebrovascular accident: Damage to the blood vessels of the cerebrum, leading to loss of blood supply to brain tissue; a **stroke.**

Concussion: Brief loss of consciousness as a result of injury to the brain.

Epilepsy: Chronic brain disorder characterized by recurrent **seizure** activity.

Glioblastoma: Malignant brain tumor arising from **glial cells.** BLAST- means immature.

Hemiplegia: **Paralysis** (-PLEGIA) that affects the right or left half of the body.

Meningitis: Inflammation of the **meninges** (membranes surrounding the brain and spinal cord).

Multiple sclerosis: Destruction of the **myelin sheath** on nerve cells in the central nervous system (brain and spinal cord), with replacement by plaques of sclerotic (hard) tissue.

Paraplegia: **Paralysis** that affects the lower portion of the body. From the Greek, meaning "to strike" (-PLEGIA) on one side (PARA-). This term was previously used to describe **hemiplegia.**

Syncope: Fainting; sudden and temporary loss of consciousness as a result of inadequate flow of blood to the brain.

VIII. NERVOUS SYSTEM (Continued)

Laboratory Tests and Diagnostic Procedures

Consult *Appendix II* for pronunciation of terms and additional information.

Cerebral angiography: X-ray imaging of the blood vessels in the brain after the injection of contrast material into an artery.

Cerebrospinal fluid (CSF) analysis: Chemical tests (for sodium, chloride, protein, and glucose), cell counts, cultures, and bacterial smears on samples of CSF to detect diseases of the brain or meninges. A lumbar puncture is used to remove CSF for analysis.

Computed tomography (CT scan):   Cross-sectional x-ray images of the brain and spinal cord (with and without contrast).

Electroencephalography (EEG):   The recording of the electrical activity within the brain.

Lumbar puncture (LP):   Pressure of CSF is measured and contrast may be injected for imaging **(myelography)** after removal of CSF from a space between the lumbar vertebrae. An LP or a spinal tap also provides a sample of cerebrospinal fluid for analysis.

Magnetic resonance imaging (MRI):   Magnetic waves and radiofrequency waves are used to create an image of the brain and spinal cord.

Positron emission tomography (PET scan):   Uptake of radioactive material in the brain shows how the brain uses glucose and gives information about brain function.

Treatment Procedures

Stereotactic radiosurgery: Placement of the skull of a stereotactic instrument that locates a target (such as a tumor) in the brain. Then a high-energy radiation beam (gamma knife) is delivered to that precise target to destroy the tissue.

Transcutaneous electrical nerve stimulation (TENS):   A battery-powered device delivers stimulation to nerves to relieve acute and chronic pain.

Matching Exercises

The following exercises will help you review terminology related to the nervous system. Answers are found on pp. 277-278.

A. Match the term in Column I with its description in Column II.

Column I		Column II
1. cerebrum	_C_	A. Lower part of the brain, nearest to the spinal cord; it controls breathing and heart beat
2. spinal cord	_B_	
3. cerebellum	_E_	B. Collection of nerves that are within the spinal cavity, surrounded by backbones
4. medulla oblongata	_A_	
5. spinal nerves	_D_	C. Largest part of the brain; controls body movements, thought, reasoning, vision, hearing, speech
		D. Nerves that transmit messages to and from the spinal cord
		E. Lower back part of the brain that controls muscular coordination and balance

B. Match the combining form in Column I with its meaning in Column II.

Column I		Column II
1. cerebell/o	_B_	A. Nerve
2. medull/o	_E_	B. Cerebellum
3. myel/o	_D_	C. Brain
4. cerebr/o	_F_	D. Spinal cord
5. encephal/o	_C_	E. Medulla oblongata
6. neur/o	_A_	F. Cerebrum

VIII. NERVOUS SYSTEM (Continued)

C. Match the medical term in Column I with its meaning in Column II.

Column I		Column II
1. myelitis	_D_	A. Disease of nerves
2. cerebral	_B_	B. Pertaining to the largest part of the brain
3. medullary	_F_	C. Pertaining to the posterior portion of the brain that controls equilibrium
4. encephalitis	_E_	
5. neuropathy	_A_	D. Inflammation of the spinal cord
6. cerebellar	_C_	E. Inflammation of the brain
		F. Pertaining to the lower part of the brain closest to the spinal cord

D. Match the pathological term in Column I with its meaning in Column II.

Column I		Column II
1. cerebrovascular accident	_E_	A. Inflammation of the membrane surrounding the brain and spinal cord
2. multiple sclerosis	_F_	
3. concussion	_G_	B. Brain disorder marked by deterioration in mental activity (dementia)
4. syncope	_C_	C. Fainting
5. epilepsy	_J_	D. Paralysis on one side of the body
6. meningitis	_A_	E. Damage to blood vessels in the brain; a stroke
7. glioblastoma	_I_	
8. paraplegia	_H_	F. Destruction of myelin sheath around nerve cells in the CNS
9. hemiplegia	_D_	G. Brief loss of consciousness from injury to the brain
10. Alzheimer disease	_B_	

H. Paralysis of the lower portion of the body

I. Malignant tumor of the brain

J. Chronic brain disorder with seizure activity

E. Match the test or procedure in Column I with its description in Column II.

Column I		Column II
1. lumbar puncture	_D_	A. Uptake of radioactive material in the brain shows how the brain uses glucose
2. CSF analysis	_B_	
3. cerebral angiography	_E_	B. Chemical tests, cell counts, cultures, and smears of fluid surrounding the brain and spinal cord
4. electroencephalogram	_C_	
5. PET scan	_A_	C. Record of the electrical activity in the brain
6. MRI	_H_	D. Procedure to remove cerebrospinal fluid; measurement of pressure and injection of contrast
7. stereotactic radiosurgery	_I_	
8. CT scan	_G_	E. X-ray image of blood vessels in the brain after injection of contrast
9. TENS	_F_	

F. A battery-powered device delivers stimulation to nerves to relieve acute and chronic pain

G. Cross-sectional x-ray images of the brain and spinal cord

H. Magnetic and radio waves create images of the brain and spinal cord tissue

I. Gamma knife is used to destroy brain tissue after a lesion is located with a special instrument

IX. RESPIRATORY SYSTEM

Anatomy

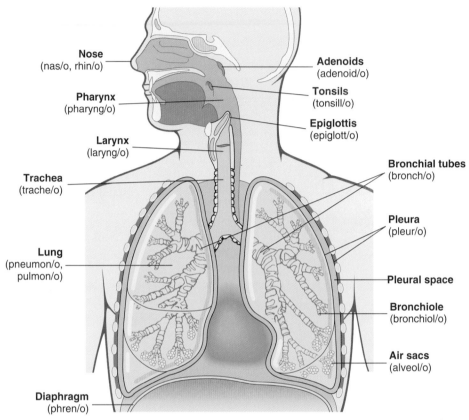

Air enters the nose and travels to the pharynx (throat). From the pharynx, air passes through the epiglottis and larynx (voice box) into the trachea (windpipe). The trachea splits into two tubes, the bronchial tubes, that carry air into the lungs. The bronchial tubes divide into smaller tubes called bronchioles that end in small air sacs. Thin air sacs allow oxygen to pass through them into tiny capillaries containing red blood cells. Red blood cells transport the oxygen to all parts of the body. In a similar manner, gaseous waste (carbon dioxide) leaves the blood by entering air sacs and traveling out of the body through bronchioles, bronchial tubes, trachea, larynx, pharynx, and the nose. (Modified from Chabner D-E: *The Language of Medicine,* ed 7, Philadelphia, 2004, WB Saunders.)

Terminology

Meanings for terminology are found in the *Glossary of Medical Terms.*

Combining Form	Meaning	Terminology	Meaning
adenoid/o	adenoid	adenoidectomy	
alveol/o	air sac; alveolus	alveolar	
bronch/o	bronchial tube	bronchoscopy	
bronchiol/o	bronchiole	bronchiolitis	
cyan/o	blue	cyanosis	
epiglott/o	epiglottis	epiglottitis	
laryng/o	larynx	laryngeal	
nas/o	nose	nasal	
rhin/o	nose	rhinorrhea	
pharyng/o	pharynx	pharyngitis	
phren/o	diaphragm	phrenic	
pneumon/o	lung	pneumonectomy	
pulmon/o	lung	pulmonary	
tonsill/o	tonsils	tonsillitis	
trache/o	trachea	tracheostomy	

IX. RESPIRATORY SYSTEM (Continued)

Pathology

Definitions for additional terms in boldface are found in the *Glossary of Medical Terms.*

Asphyxia: Extreme decrease in the amount of **oxygen** in the body with increase of **carbon dioxide** leads to loss of consciousness or death.

Asthma: Spasm and narrowing of bronchi, leading to bronchial airway obstruction.

Atelectasis: Collapsed lung (ATEL/O- means incomplete, and -ECTASIS indicates dilation or expansion).

Emphysema: Hyperinflation of air sacs with destruction of alveolar walls. Along with chronic **bronchitis** and **asthma,** emphysema is a type of **chronic obstructive pulmonary disease.**

Hemoptysis: Spitting up of blood.

Hemothorax: Blood in the pleural cavity (space between the **pleura**).

Pneumoconiosis: Abnormal condition of dust (CONI/O-) in the lungs.

Pneumonia: Inflammation and infection of alveoli, which fill with pus or products of the inflammatory reaction.

Tuberculosis: An infectious disease caused by bacteria (bacilli). The lungs and other organs are affected. Symptoms are cough, weight loss, night sweats, **hemoptysis,** and pleuritic pain.

Laboratory Test and Diagnostic Procedures

Consult *Appendix II* for pronunciation of terms and additional information.

Bronchoscopy: Visual examination of the bronchial tubes with an endoscope.

Chest x-ray film: X-ray image of the chest in the A/P (antero-posterior), P/A (postero-anterior), and lateral (side) views.

Computed tomography (CT scan):   Cross-sectional x-ray images of the chest.

Laryngoscopy: Visual examination of the larynx via the placement of a flexible tube (laryngoscope) through the nose or mouth and into the larynx.

Magnetic resonance imaging (MRI):   Magnetic waves and radiofrequency waves create images of the chest in three planes of the body.

Pulmonary angiography: X-ray images are taken of the blood vessels in the lung after the injection of contrast material into a blood vessel. A blockage, such as a pulmonary embolism, can be located with this procedure.

Pulmonary function tests (PFTs):   Measurement of the ventilation (breathing capability) of the lungs (air movement in and out of the lungs). A spirometer measures the air taken in and out of the lungs.

Pulmonary ventilation and perfusion scans: Procedures that show air flow (ventilation) and blood supply (perfusion) to the lungs via the distribution of radioactive material in the lung tissue after the radioactive material is intravenously injected or is inhaled.

Sputum test: A patient expels sputum by coughing and the sputum is analyzed for bacterial content.

Tuberculin test: Agents are applied to the skin with punctures or injection and the reaction is noted. Redness and swelling result in people sensitive to the test substance and indicate prior or present infection with **tuberculosis.**

Treatment Procedures

Endotracheal intubation: A tube is placed through the nose or mouth into the trachea to establish an airway during surgery and for placement on a respirator (a machine that moves air in and out of the lungs).

Thoracentesis: A needle is inserted through the skin between the ribs and into the pleural space to drain a **pleural effusion.**

Thoracotomy: Incision of the chest to remove a lung **(pneumonectomy)** or a portion of a lung **(lobectomy).**

Tracheostomy: Creation of an opening into the trachea through the neck and the insertion of a tube to create an airway.

IX. RESPIRATORY SYSTEM (Continued)

Matching Exercises

The following exercises will help you review terminology related to the respiratory system. Answers are found on p. 278.

A. Match the term in Column I with its description in Column II.

Column I		Column II
1. nose	F	A. Throat
2. epiglottis	D	B. Windpipe
3. larynx	I	C. Muscle that separates the chest from the abdomen
4. pharynx	A	
5. lung	J	D. Flap of cartilage over the mouth of the trachea
6. diaphragm	C	E. Small bronchial tube
7. trachea	B	F. Structure on the face that permits air to enter the body
8. bronchial tube	H	
9. bronchiole	E	G. Thin-walled sac through which gases can pass into and out of the bloodstream
10. air sac	G	H. One of two tubes that carry air from the windpipe to the lungs
		I. Voice box
		J. One of two paired organs in the chest through which oxygen enters and carbon dioxide leaves the bloodstream

B. Match the combining form in Column I with its meaning in Column II.

Column I		Column II
1. pharyng/o	E	A. Diaphragm

2. bronch/o _G_   B. Air sac

3. bronchiol/o _I_   C. Windpipe

4. nas/o or rhin/o _D_   D. Nose

5. laryng/o _F_   E. Throat

6. phren/o _A_   F. Voice box

7. trache/o _C_   G. Tube that carries air from the windpipe to the lung

8. epiglott/o _J_

9. alveol/o _B_   H. Lung

10. pneumon/o _H_   I. Small bronchus

J. Epiglottis

C. Match the medical term in Column I with its meaning in Column II.

Column I		Column II
1. pulmonary	_D_	A. Discharge from the nose
2. rhinorrhea	_A_	B. Pertaining to an air sac
3. pneumonectomy	_H_	C. Inflammation of the throat
4. bronchoscopy	_G_	D. Pertaining to a lung
5. laryngeal	_I_	E. New opening of the windpipe to the outside of the body
6. pharyngitis	_C_	F. Pertaining to the nose
7. phrenic	_J_	G. Visual examination of the bronchus
8. tracheostomy	_E_	H. Resection of a lung
9. alveolar	_B_	I. Pertaining to the voice box
10. nasal	_F_	J. Pertaining to the diaphragm

IX. RESPIRATORY SYSTEM (Continued)

D. Match the pathological term in Column I with its meaning in Column II.

Column I		Column II
1. atelectasis	A	A. Collapsed lung
2. hemothorax	F	B. Condition of dust particles in the lung
3. asphyxia	G	C. Spitting up blood
4. emphysema	H	D. Infectious disease caused by bacilli; lungs and other organs are affected
5. asthma	I	
6. hemoptysis	C	E. Inflammation and infection of alveoli
7. tuberculosis	D	F. Blood in the pleural space
8. pneumonia	E	G. Extreme decrease in oxygen and increase in carbon dioxide in the blood
9. pneumoconiosis	B	H. Hyperinflation of air sacs and destruction of alveolar walls
		I. Spasm and narrowing of bronchial tubes leading to airway obstruction

E. Match the test or procedure in Column I with its description in Column II.

Column I		Column II
1. pulmonary angiography	G	A. X-ray image in A/P, P/A, or lateral view
2. laryngoscopy	H	B. Material expelled by coughing is analyzed
3. pulmonary ventilation and perfusion scans	D	C. Visual examination of bronchial tubes
4. PFTs	F	D. After injecting or inhaling radioactive material, images reveal distribution in lung tissue

5. chest x-ray   _A_

6. bronchoscopy   _C_

7. sputum test   _B_

8. MRI   _E_

9. tuberculin test   _J_

10. chest CT scan   _I_

E. Magnetic waves produce images of the chest in three planes

F. Measurements of the ventilation capability of the lung using a spirometer

G. X-ray images of blood vessels in the lung

H. Visual examination of the voice box

I. Cross-sectional x-ray images of the chest

J. Agents are applied to the skin with punctures, and reaction is noted

F. **Match the treatment procedure in Column I with its description in Column II.**

Column I	Column II
1. tracheostomy _B_	A. A tube placed through the nose or mouth into the windpipe to establish an airway
2. thoracentesis _D_	B. Creation of an opening into the windpipe through the neck and insertion of a tube to create an airway
3. endotracheal intubation _A_	C. Incision of the chest to remove a lung or a portion of a lung
4. thoracotomy _C_	D. Insertion of a needle through the skin between the ribs and into the pleural space to drain a pleural effusion

X. SKIN AND SENSE ORGANS

Anatomy

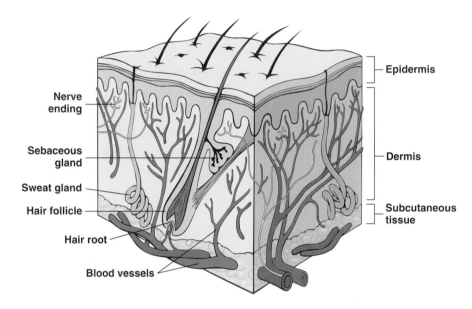

Skin (derm/o, dermat/o, cutane/o)

Epidermis

Dermis

Subcutaneous tissue

Nerve ending

Sebaceous gland

Sweat gland

Hair follicle

Hair root

Blood vessels

Eye
(ophthalm/o, ocul/o)

Retina (retin/o)

Optic nerve

Sclera

Conjunctiva

Cornea

Lens (phak/o)

Pupil

Path of light

Iris

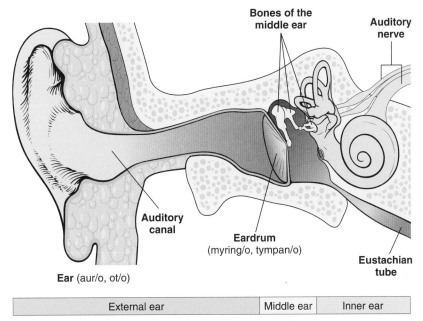

The skin and sense organs receive messages (touch sensations, light waves, sound waves) from the environment and send them to the brain via nerves. These messages are interpreted in the brain, making sight, hearing, and perception of the environment possible. (Modified from Chabner D-E: *The Language of Medicine,* ed 7, Philadelphia, 2004, WB Saunders.)

X. SKIN AND SENSE ORGANS (Continued)

Terminology

Meanings for terminology are found in the *Glossary of Medical Terms*.

Combining Form	Meaning	Terminology	Meaning
aur/o	ear	aural discharge _____	
ot/o	ear	otitis _____	
cutane/o	skin	subcutaneous _____	
derm/o	skin	epidermis _____	
dermat/o	skin	dermatology _____	
myring/o	eardrum	myringotomy _____	
tympan/o	eardrum	tympanoplasty _____	
ocul/o	eye	ocular _____	
ophthalm/o	eye	ophthalmoscope _____	
phak/o	lens of the eye	aphakia _____	
retin/o	retina	retinopathy _____	

Pathology

Definitions for additional terms in boldface are found in the *Glossary of Medical Terms.*

Alopecia: Absence of hair from areas where it normally grows; baldness.

Cataract: Clouding (opacity) of the lens of the eye, causing impairment of vision or blindness.

Conjunctivitis: Inflammation of the **conjunctiva.**

Glaucoma: Increase in pressure (fluid accumulation) within the chamber at the front of the eye.

Melanoma: Malignant tumor of pigmented cells (MELAN/O- means black) that arises from a **nevus** (mole) in the skin.

Nevus: Pigmented lesion in or on the skin; a mole.

Tinnitus: Abnormal noise (ringing, buzzing, roaring) sound in the ears.

Laboratory Tests and Diagnostic Procedures

Consult *Appendix II* for pronunciation of terms and additional information.

Allergy test: Procedure in which allergy-causing substances are placed on the skin and a reaction is noted. In the patch test, a patch with a suspected allergen is placed on the skin. The scratch test involves making several scratches and the insertion of a small amount of allergen in the scratches.

Bacterial and fungal tests: Procedures in which samples from skin lesions are taken to determine the presence of bacterial infection or fungal growth.

Fluorescein angiography: Fluorescein (a contrast) is injected intravenously and the movement of blood is observed by ophthalmoscopy. It is used to detect diabetic or hypertensive retinopathy and also degeneration of the macular (central) area of the retina.

Ophthalmoscopy: Visual examination of the interior of the eye.

Otoscopy: Visual examination of the ear (to the eardrum).

Skin biopsy: Procedure in which skin lesions are removed and sent to the pathology laboratory for microscopic examination.

Slit-lamp microscopy: Procedure in which the anterior eye structures (such as the cornea) are microscopically examined with an instrument called a slit lamp.

Tuning fork tests: Procedure in which a vibration source (tuning fork) is placed in front of the opening to the ear to test air conduction of sound waves. The tuning fork is also placed on the mastoid bone behind the ear to test bone conduction of sound waves.

X. SKIN AND SENSE ORGANS (Continued)

Matching Exercises

The following exercises will help you review terminology related to the skin and sense organs. Answers are found on pp. 278-279.

A. Match the term in Column I with its description in Column II.

Column I		Column II
1. epidermis	E	A. Oil-producing gland in the skin
2. sebaceous gland	A	B. Gland in the skin that produces a watery, salt-containing fluid
3. dermis	D	C. Innermost layer of the skin, composed of fatty tissue
4. subcutaneous tissue	C	D. Middle layer of the skin, containing hair follicles, connective tissue, blood vessels, and glands
5. sweat gland	B	E. Outer layer of the skin

B. Match the term in Column I with its description in Column II.

Column I		Column II
1. retina	G	A. White, outer coat of the eyeball
2. conjunctiva	K	B. Membrane that separates the outer and middle parts of the ear
3. pupil	F	C. Transparent structure behind the pupil that bends light rays so that they focus on the back of the eye
4. lens	C	D. Nerve that carries messages from the inner ear to the brain
5. cornea	E	
6. sclera	A	

7. iris   _I_

8. eardrum   _B_

9. auditory canal   _J_

10. auditory nerve   _D_

11. optic nerve   _H_

E. Transparent layer over the front of the eye that bends light that bends light so that it is focused on the back of the eye

F. Black center of the eye through which light enters

G. Layer of sensitive cells at the back of the eye

H. Nerve at the back of the eye that transmits light waves to the brain

I. Colored, pigmented portion of the eye

J. Passageway leading into the ear from the outside of the body

K. Thin, protective membrane over the front of the eye

C. Match the combining form in Column I with its meaning in Column II.

Column I		Column II
1. derm/o	_C_	A. Eye
2. phak/o	_E_	B. Ear
3. retin/o	_D_	C. Skin
4. myring/o	_F_	D. Posterior, sensitive cell layer of the eye
5. aur/o	_B_	E. Lens of the eye
6. ophthalm/o	_A_	F. Eardrum

X. SKIN AND SENSE ORGANS (Continued)

D. Match the medical term in Column I with its meaning in Column II.

Column I		Column II
1. ocular	_E_	A. Disease of the rod and cone layer of eye (sensitive cells at the back of the eye)
2. otitis	_D_	B. Surgical repair of the eardrum
3. subcutaneous	_F_	C. Absence of the lens of the eye
4. myringotomy	_G_	D. Inflammation of the ear
5. aphakia	_C_	E. Pertaining to the eye
6. epidermis	_H_	F. Pertaining to under the skin
7. retinopathy	_A_	G. Incision of the eardrum
8. ophthalmoscope	_I_	H. Outer layer of the skin
9. tympanoplasty	_B_	I. Instrument to visually examine the eye

E. Match the pathological term in Column I with its meaning in Column II.

Column I		Column II
1. melanoma	_F_	A. Clouding of the lens of the eye, causing impairment of vision
2. glaucoma	_D_	B. Absence of hair from areas where it normally grows
3. conjunctivitis	_G_	C. Pigmented lesion on the skin; mole
4. tinnitus	_E_	D. Increase in pressure within the chamber at the front of the eye
5. cataract	_A_	E. Abnormal noise (ringing, buzzing) or sound in the ears
6. nevus	_C_	
7. alopecia	_B_	

F. Malignant tumor of pigmented cells in the skin

G. Inflammation of the mucous membrane lining the inner surface of the eyelid

F. Match the test or procedure in Column I with its description in Column II.

Column I		Column II
1. skin biopsy	D	A. Samples from skin lesions are examined to detect presence of microorganisms
2. slit-lamp microscopy	G	
3. tuning fork tests	H	B. Visual examination of the interior of the eye
4. fluorescein angiography	E	C. Patch test; scratch test
5. otoscopy	F	D. Skin lesions are removed and sent for pathologic microscope examination
6. allergy test	C	
7. bacterial and fungal tests	A	E. A dye is injected intravenously, and movement of blood through blood vessels in the back of the eye is observed with an ophthalmoscope
8. ophthalmoscopy	B	

F. Visual examination of the ear to the eardrum

G. Examination of the anterior eye structures, such as the cornea, under a microscope

H. A vibration source is placed in front of the opening of the ear to test air conduction of sound waves

XI. URINARY SYSTEM

Anatomy

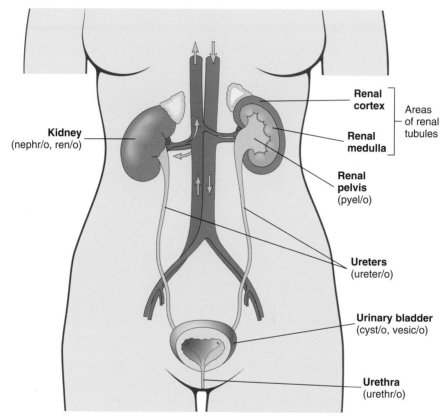

Renal
cortex
⎤
⎥ Areas
⎥ of renal
⎥ tubules
Renal
medulla
⎦

Kidney
(nephr/o, ren/o)

Renal
pelvis
(pyel/o)

Ureters
(ureter/o)

Urinary bladder
(cyst/o, vesic/o)

Urethra
(urethr/o)

Urine is formed as waste materials, such as urea, are filtered from the blood into the tubules of the kidney. Urine passes from the tubules into the central collecting section of the kidney, the renal pelvis. Each renal pelvis leads directly to a ureter, which takes the urine to the urinary bladder. The bladder releases urine to the urethra and urine leaves the body. (Modified from Chabner D-E: *The Language of Medicine,* ed 7, Philadelphia, 2004, WB Saunders.)

Terminology

Meanings for terminology are found in the *Glossary of Medical Terms*.

Combining Form	Meaning	Terminology	Meaning
cyst/o	urinary bladder	cystoscopy _____	
vesic/o	urinary bladder	vesical _____	
nephr/o	kidney	nephritis _____	
ren/o	kidney	renal _____	
pyel/o	renal pelvis	pyelogram _____	
ureter/o	ureter	ureterectomy _____	
urethr/o	urethra	urethritis _____	

Pathology

Definitions for additional terms in boldface are found in the *Glossary of Medical Terms*.

Albuminuria: Abnormal condition of protein (albumin) in the urine.
Anuria: Abnormal condition of no urine production.
Dysuria: Painful urination.
Glycosuria: Abnormal condition of glucose in the urine.
Hematuria: Abnormal condition of blood in the urine.
Nephrolithiasis: Abnormal condition of stones in the kidney.
Renal failure: Condition in which the kidneys stop functioning and do not produce urine.
Uremia: Condition of high levels of **urea** (nitrogenous waste material) in the blood.

XI. URINARY SYSTEM (Continued)

Laboratory Tests and Diagnostic Procedures

Consult *Appendix II* for pronunciation of terms and additional information.

Blood urea nitrogen (BUN):   Measures the amount of **urea** (nitrogenous waste) in the blood.

Cystoscopy: Visual examination of the urinary bladder with a **cystoscope** (endoscope).

Kidneys, ureters, bladder (KUB):   X-ray image of the kidneys and urinary tract without the use of contrast.

Intravenous pyelogram (IVP):   Contrast material is injected intravenously and x-ray images are taken of the urinary tract (kidneys, ureters, bladder, and urethra). Also called **urography.**

Retrograde pyelogram (RP):   Contrast material injected via a catheter (a flexible, tubular instrument) into the urethra and bladder and x-ray films taken of the urethra, bladder, and ureters. Also called **urography.**

Voiding cystourethrogram (VCUG):   X-ray films of the bladder and urethra taken after the bladder is filled with a contrast material and while a patient is expelling urine. Also called **cystography.**

Treatment Procedures

Dialysis: Waste materials (**urea, creatinine,** and uric acid) are separated from the blood by a machine (**hemodialysis**). Alternatively, a peritoneal catheter (a flexible, tubular instrument) delivers a special fluid into the abdominal cavity, and then a fluid, which contains waste materials that have seeped from the blood into it, is drained (**peritoneal dialysis**).

Extracorporeal shock wave lithotripsy (ESWL):   Shock waves are beamed into a patient to crush urinary tract stones. The stone fragments then pass out of the body with urine. Also called **lithotripsy.**

Renal transplantation: A donor kidney is transferred to a recipient.

Urinary catheterization: A catheter (a flexible, tubular instrument) is passed through the urethra and into the urinary bladder for short-term or long-term drainage of urine.

Matching Exercises

The following exercises will help you review terminology related to the urinary system.
Answers are found on p. 279.

A. Match the term in Column I with its description in Column II.

Column I	Column II
1. urinary bladder _____	A. Tube that leads from the bladder to the outside of the body
2. kidney _____	B. Central section of the kidney
3. renal pelvis _____	C. Organ behind the abdomen that makes urine by filtering wastes from the blood
4. ureter _____	D. One of two tubes that carry urine from the kidney to the urinary bladder
5. urethra _____	E. Muscular sac that holds urine and releases it to leave the body through the urethra

B. Match the combining form in Column I with its meaning in Column II.

Column I	Column II
1. ureter/o _____	A. Urinary bladder
2. urethr/o _____	B. Tube leading from the urinary bladder to the outside of the body
3. pyel/o _____	C. Kidney
4. cyst/o, vesic/o _____	D. Tube leading from the kidney to the urinary bladder
5. nephr/o, ren/o _____	E. Renal pelvis (central collecting basin of the kidney)

XI. URINARY SYSTEM (Continued)

C. Match the medical term in Column I with its meaning in Column II.

Column I		Column II
1. pyelogram	_____	A. X-ray record of the renal pelvis
2. urethritis	_____	B. Visual examination of the urinary bladder
3. nephritis	_____	C. Resection of a ureter
4. vesical	_____	D. Pertaining to the urinary bladder
5. cystoscopy	_____	E. Inflammation of the kidney
6. ureterectomy	_____	F. Pertaining to the kidney
7. renal	_____	G. Inflammation of the urethra

D. Match the pathological term in Column I with its meaning in Column II.

Column I		Column II
1. dysuria	_____	A. Kidneys stop functioning and fail to produce urine
2. hematuria	_____	
3. uremia	_____	B. Abnormal condition of protein in urine
4. renal failure	_____	C. Blood in the urine
5. nephrolithiasis	_____	D. No urine production
6. albuminuria	_____	E. High levels of urea in the bloodstream
7. glycosuria	_____	F. Sugar in the urine
8. anuria	_____	G. Painful urination
		H. Abnormal condition of kidney stones

E. Match the test or procedure in Column I with its description in Column II.

Column I	Column II
1. KUB _____	A. Measurement of amount of nitrogenous wastes in the blood
2. dialysis _____	
	B. Visual examination of the urinary bladder
3. VCUG _____	
	C. X-ray image of the kidneys and urinary tract without contrast
4. ESWL _____	
5. renal transplantation _____	D. Tube is passed through the urethra into the urinary bladder for short- or long-term drainage of urine
6. cystoscopy _____	
7. BUN _____	E. Shock waves are beamed into the patient to crush stones in the kidney or ureter
8. retrograde pyelogram _____	F. Nitrogenous waste materials are separated from the blood by a machine
9. IVP _____	
10. urinary catheterization _____	G. Contrast material is injected intravenously, and x-ray images are taken of the bladder as the patient is expelling urine
	H. After filling the bladder with contrast, x-ray images are taken of the bladder as the patient is expelling urine
	I. Contrast material is injected via a catheter into the bladder, and x-ray images are taken of the ureters, bladder, and urethra
	J. A kidney from a donor is surgically implanted in a patient whose kidneys have failed

Answers to Matching Exercises

I. CARDIOVASCULAR SYSTEM

A

1. B	3. F	5. D	7. J	9. C
2. I	4. E	6. A	8. G	10. H

B

1. D	2. E	3. B	4. F	5. A	6. C

C

1. D	3. G	5. H	7. A
2. F	4. C	6. E	8. B

D

1. E	3. D	5. C	7. F
2. H	4. G	6. A	8. B

E

1. I	3. C	5. B	7. D	9. H
2. J	4. G	6. E	8. A	10. F

F

1. E	2. B	3. D	4. F	5. A	6. C

II. DIGESTIVE SYSTEM

A

1. G	3. H	5. F	7. B
2. C	4. A	6. D	8. E

B

1. C	3. A	5. D	7. G
2. H	4. F	6. B	8. E

C

1. D	3. H	5. J	7. E	9. C
2. G	4. I	6. A	8. F	10. B

D

1. C	3. G	5. D	7. J	9. A
2. F	4. H	6. I	8. E	10. B

E

| 1. D | 3. E | 5. A | 7. B |
| 2. F | 4. G | 6. C | |

F

| 1. G | 3. A | 5. C | 7. J | 9. E |
| 2. I | 4. D | 6. H | 8. F | 10. B |

III. ENDOCRINE SYSTEM

A

| 1. C | 3. A | 5. G | 7. F |
| 2. H | 4. E | 6. B | 8. D |

B

| 1. F | 3. E | 5. H | 7. B |
| 2. D | 4. G | 6. C | 8. A |

C

| 1. D | 3. F | 5. G | 7. A |
| 2. H | 4. B | 6. E | 8. C |

D

| 1. C | 2. D | 3. A | 4. B | 5. E |

E

| 1. B | 3. A | 5. F | 7. D |
| 2. E | 4. G | 6. C | |

IV. FEMALE REPRODUCTIVE SYSTEM

A

| 1. C | 2. B | 3. D | 4. A | 5. F | 6. E |

B

| 1. D | 2. E | 3. B | 4. A | 5. C | 6. F |

C

| 1. D | 3. H | 5. G | 7. E |
| 2. F | 4. A | 6. B | 8. C |

D

| 1. C | 3. D | 5. A | 7. B |
| 2. E | 4. G | 6. F | |

E

| 1. H | 3. C | 5. D | 7. E | 9. I |
| 2. F | 4. A | 6. G | 8. B | |

F

| 1. C | 2. A | 3. E | 4. B | 5. D |

V. LYMPHATIC SYSTEM

A

| 1. C | 2. B | 3. D | 4. A | 5. E |

B

| 1. C | 2. D | 3. E | 4. A | 5. B |

C

| 1. G | 3. E | 5. F | 7. C |
| 2. D | 4. A | 6. B | |

D

| 1. D | 2. C | 3. E | 4. B | 5. A |

VI. MALE REPRODUCTIVE SYSTEM

A

| 1. C | 2. B | 3. D | 4. A | 5. E |

B

| 1. B | 2. E | 3. D | 4. F | 5. C | 6. A |

C

| 1. D | 3. F | 5. A | 7. B |
| 2. E | 4. C | 6. G | |

D

| 1. E | 2. F | 3. C | 4. D | 5. B | 6. A |

E

| 1. E | 2. F | 3. D | 4. C | 5. A | 6. B |

VII. MUSCULOSKELETAL SYSTEM

A

1. H	5. J	9. T	13. L	17. F
2. E	6. R	10. G	14. P	18. M
3. K	7. Q	11. I	15. C	19. B
4. D	8. A	12. S	16. N	20. O

B

| 1. D | 3. H | 5. G | 7. I | 9. A |
| 2. C | 4. E | 6. F | 8. B | 10. J |

C

| 1. G | 3. D | 5. B | 7. C | 9. A |
| 2. E | 4. I | 6. F | 8. H | |

D

| 1. C | 2. B | 3. E | 4. F | 5. A | 6. D |

E

| 1. E | 3. A | 5. B | 7. D | 9. J |
| 2. G | 4. F | 6. C | 8. I | 10. H |

F

| 1. D | 2. C | 3. A | 4. B | 5. E |

VIII. NERVOUS SYSTEM

A

| 1. C | 2. B | 3. E | 4. A | 5. D |

B

| 1. B | 2. E | 3. D | 4. F | 5. C | 6. A |

C

| 1. D | 2. B | 3. F | 4. E | 5. A | 6. C |

D

| 1. E | 3. G | 5. J | 7. I | 9. D |
| 2. F | 4. C | 6. A | 8. H | 10. B |

E

| 1. D | 3. E | 5. A | 7. I | 9. F |
| 2. B | 4. C | 6. H | 8. G | |

IX. RESPIRATORY SYSTEM

A

| 1. F | 3. I | 5. J | 7. B | 9. E |
| 2. D | 4. A | 6. C | 8. H | 10. G |

B

| 1. E | 3. I | 5. F | 7. C | 9. B |
| 2. G | 4. D | 6. A | 8. J | 10. H |

C

| 1. D | 3. H | 5. I | 7. J | 9. B |
| 2. A | 4. G | 6. C | 8. E | 10. F |

D

| 1. A | 3. G | 5. I | 7. D | 9. B |
| 2. F | 4. H | 6. C | 8. E | |

E

| 1. G | 3. D | 5. A | 7. B | 9. J |
| 2. H | 4. F | 6. C | 8. E | 10. I |

F

| 1. B | 2. D | 3. A | 4. C |

X. SKIN AND SENSE ORGANS

A

| 1. E | 2. A | 3. D | 4. C | 5. B |

B

| 1. G | 3. F | 5. E | 7. I | 9. J | 11. H |
| 2. K | 4. C | 6. A | 8. B | 10. D | |

C

| 1. C | 2. E | 3. D | 4. F | 5. B | 6. A |

D

1. E	3. F	5. C	7. A	9. B
2. D	4. G	6. H	8. I	

E

1. F	3. G	5. A	7. B
2. D	4. E	6. C	

F

1. D	3. H	5. F	7. A
2. G	4. E	6. C	8. B

XI. URINARY SYSTEM

A

1. E	2. C	3. B	4. D	5. A

B

1. D	2. B	3. E	4. A	5. C

C

1. A	3. E	5. B	7. F
2. G	4. D	6. C	

D

1. G	3. E	5. H	7. F
2. C	4. A	6. B	8. D

E

1. C	3. H	5. J	7. A	9. G
2. F	4. E	6. B	8. I	10. D

Diagnostic Tests and Procedures*

*This appendix also appears in the CD-ROM in this format and as a complete alphabetical reference.

RADIOLOGY, ULTRASOUND, AND IMAGING PROCEDURES

In many of the following procedures, a *contrast* substance (sometimes referred to as a *dye*) is introduced into or around a body part so that the part can be viewed while x-rays are taken. The contrast substance (often containing barium or iodine) appears dense on the x-ray and outlines the body part that it fills.

The suffix -GRAPHY, meaning "process of recording," is used in many terms describing imaging procedures. The suffix -GRAM, meaning "record," is also used and describes the actual image that is produced by this procedure.

Pronunciation of each term is given with its meaning. The syllable that gets the accent is in CAPITAL LETTERS. *Italicized* terms indicate important additional terminology, and terms in SMALL CAPITAL LETTERS are defined elsewhere in this appendix.

Angiography (an-je-OG-rah-fe) or **angiogram** (AN-je-o-gram): X-ray imaging of blood vessels. A contrast substance is injected into blood vessels (veins and arteries), and x-ray images are taken of the vessels. In *cerebral angiography,* x-ray images show blood vessels in the brain. In *coronary angiography,* x-rays detect abnormalities in vessels that bring blood to the heart. Angiograms can detect blockage by clots, cholesterol plaques, or tumors or aneurysms (ballooning or dilating of the vessel wall). Angiography is performed most frequently to view arteries and is often used interchangeably with *arteriography.*

Arteriography (ar-ter-e-OG-rah-fe) or **arteriogram** (ar-TER-e-oh-gram): X-ray recording of arteries after injection of a contrast substance into an artery. *Coronary arteriography* is the visualization of arteries that travel across the outer surface of the heart and bring blood to the heart muscle.

Arthrography (arth-ROG-ra-Fe): X-ray examination of the inside of a joint with a contrast medium.

Barium tests (BAH-re-um tests): X-ray examinations with a liquid barium mixture to locate disorders in the esophagus *(esophagogram),* duodenum, small intestine *(small bowel follow-through),* and colon *(barium enema).* Taken before or during the examination, barium causes the intestinal tract to stand out in silhouette when viewed through a *fluoroscope* or seen on an x-ray film. The *barium swallow* is used to examine the upper gastrointestinal tract, and the *barium enema* is for examination of the lower gastrointestinal tract.

Barium enema: See LOWER GASTROINTESTINAL EXAMINATION and BARIUM TESTS.

Barium swallow: See ESOPHAGOGRAPHY, BARIUM TESTS, and UPPER GI SERIES.

Bone density test (bon-DEN-se-te test): Low-energy x-rays reveal areas of bone deficiency *(osteopenia)* and *osteoporosis.*

Cardiac catheterization (KAR-de-ak cath-eh-ter-i-ZA-shun): Procedure in which a catheter (tube) is passed via vein or artery into the chambers of the heart to measure the blood flow out of the heart and the pressures and oxygen content in the heart chambers. Contrast material is also introduced into heart chambers, and x-ray images are taken to show heart structure.

Cerebral angiography: See ANGIOGRAPHY.

Chest x-ray: An x-ray of the chest wall, lungs, and heart. It may show infection (as in pneumonia or tuberculosis), emphysema, occupational exposure (asbestosis), lung tumors, or heart enlargement.

Cholangiography (kol-an-je-OG-rah-fe) or **cholangiogram** (kol-AN-je-o-gram): X-ray recording of bile ducts. Contrast material is given by intravenous injection *(I.V. cholangiogram)* and collects in the gallbladder and bile ducts. Also, contrast can be introduced (through the skin) with a percutaneously placed needle inserted into an intrahepatic duct *(percutaneous transhepatic cholangiography)*. X-rays are taken of bile ducts to identify obstructions caused by tumors or stones.

Computed tomography (CT) (kom-PU-ted to-MOG-ra-fe):   X-ray images taken to show the body in cross-section. Contrast material may be used (injected into the bloodstream) to highlight structures such as the liver, brain, or blood vessels, and barium can be swallowed to outline gastrointestinal organs. X-ray images, taken as the x-ray tube rotates (helical CT) around the body, are processed by a computer to show "slices" of body tissues, most often within the head, chest, and abdomen.

Coronary arteriography: See ARTERIOGRAPHY.

Cystography (sis-TOG-rah-fe) or **cystogram** (SIS-to-gram):   X-ray recording of the urinary bladder with a contrast medium so that the outline of the urinary bladder can be seen clearly. A contrast substance is injected via catheter into the urethra and urinary bladder, and x-ray images are taken. A *voiding cystourethrogram* is an x-ray image of the urinary tract made while the patient is urinating.

Digital subtraction angiography (DIJ-i-tal sub-TRAK-shun an-je-OG-rah-fe):   A unique x-ray technique for viewing blood vessels by taking two images and subtracting one from the other. Images are first taken without contrast and then again after contrast is injected into blood vessels. The first image is then subtracted from the second so that the final image (sharp and precise) shows only contrast-filled blood vessels and not the surrounding tissue.

Doppler ultrasound (DOP-ler UL-tra-sound):   An instrument that focuses sound waves on blood vessels and measured blood flow as echoes bounce off red blood cells. Arteries or veins in the arms, neck, or legs are examined to detect vessels that are occluded (blocked) by clots or atherosclerosis.

Echocardiography (eh-ko-kar-de-OG-rah-fe) or **echocardiogram** (eh-ko-KAR-de-o-gram):   Images of the heart produced by introducing high-frequency sound waves through the chest into the heart. The sound waves are reflected back from the heart, and echoes showing heart structure are displayed on a recording machine. It is a highly useful diagnostic tool in the evaluation of diseases of the valves that separate the heart chambers and diseases of the heart muscle.

Endoscopic retrograde cholangiopancreatography or **ERCP** (en-do-SKOP-ik REH-tro-grad kol-an-je-o-pan-kre-ah-TOG-rah-fe):   X-ray recording of the bile ducts, pancreas, and pancreatic duct. Radiopaque contrast is injected via a tube through the mouth into the bile and pancreatic ducts, and x-rays are then taken.

Endoscopic ultrasonography or **E-US** (en-do-SKOP-ik ul-trah-so-NOG-rah-fe): Sound waves are generated from a tube inserted through the mouth and into the esophagus. The sound waves bounce off of internal structures and are detected by surface coils. E-US detects enlarged lymph nodes and tumors in the chest and upper abdomen.

Esophagography (eh-sof-ah-GOG-rah-fe) or **esophagogram** (eh-SOF-ah-go-gram): X-ray images taken of the esophagus after barium sulfate is swallowed. This test is part of a BARIUM SWALLOW and UPPER GASTROINTESTINAL EXAMINATION.

Fluoroscopy (flur-OS-ko-pe):   An x-ray procedure that uses a fluorescent screen rather than a photographic plate to show images of the body. X-rays that have passed through the body strike a screen covered with a fluorescent substance that emits yellow-green light. Internal organs are seen directly and in motion. Fluoroscopy is used to guide the insertion of catheters direct organ biopsies and may be enhanced with barium ingestion.

Gallbladder ultrasound (GAWL-blah-der UL-tra-sownd):   Sound waves are used to visualize gallstones. This procedure has replaced the x-ray test, cholecystography.

Hysterosalpingography (his-ter-o-sal-ping-OG-rah-fe) or **hysterosalpingogram** (his-ter-o-sal-PING-o-gram):   X-ray recording of the uterus and fallopian tubes. Contrast medium is inserted through the vagina into the uterus and fallopian tubes, and x-rays are taken to detect blockage or tumor.

Intravenous pyelography: See UROGRAPHY.

Kidneys, ureters, bladder (KID-nez, UR-eh-tersz, BLA-der) or **KUB:**   X-ray images of the kidney, ureters, and urinary bladder, taken without contrast.

Lower gastrointestinal examination (LO-wer gas-tro-in-TES-tin-al ek-zam-ih-NA-shun):   X-ray pictures of the colon taken after a liquid contrast substance called barium sulfate is inserted through a plastic tube (enema) into the rectum and large intestine (colon). If tumor is present in the colon, it may appear as an obstruction or irregularity. Also known as a BARIUM ENEMA.

Magnetic resonance imaging (mag-NET-ik REZ-o-nans IM-a-jing) or **MRI:** Magnetic waves, not x-rays, are used to create an image of body organs. The images can be taken in several planes of the body—frontal (coronal), sagittal (side), and transverse (axial or cross-section)—and are particularly useful for studying tumors of the brain and spinal cord and abnormalities of the chest, abdomen, and head.

Mammography (mah-MOG-rah-fe) or **mammogram** (MAM-o-gram): X-ray recording of the breast. X-rays of low voltage are beamed at the breast, and images are produced. Mammography detects abnormalities in breast tissue, such as breast cancer.

Myelography (mi-eh-LOG-rah-fe) or **myelogram** (MI-eh-lo-gram): X-ray recording of the spinal cord. This procedure is largely replaced by MRI to detect tumors or ruptured "slipped" disks between vertebrae (backbones).

Pulmonary angiography (PUL-mo-ner-e an-je-OG-rah-Fe): X-ray images taken of blood vessels of the lung after injection of contrast.

Pyelography or **pyelogram:** See UROGRAPHY.

Small bowel follow-through: See BARIUM TESTS and UPPER GASTROINTESTINAL EXAMINATION.

Tomography (to-MOG-rah-fe) or **tomogram** (TO-mo-gram): X-ray recording that shows an organ in depth. Several pictures ("slices") are taken of an organ by moving the x-ray tube and film in sequence to blur out certain regions and bring others into sharper focus. Tomograms of the kidney and lung are examples.

Ultrasonography (ul-trah-so-NOG-rah-fe) or **ultrasonogram** (ul-trah-SON-o-gram): Images produced by beaming sound waves into the body and capturing the echoes that bounce off organs. These echoes are then processed to produce an image showing the difference between fluid and solid masses and the general position of organs. Ultrasonography is particularly useful for detecting gallbladder stones, fibroid tumors of the uterus and ovarian tumors and cysts *(pelvic ultrasonography),* enlargement of the heart or defects in heart valves *(echocardiography),* and enlargement of lymph nodes in the abdomen and chest.

Upper gastrointestinal examination (UP-er gas-tro-in-TES-tin-al ek-zam-ih-NA-shun): X-ray pictures taken of the esophagus (BARIUM SWALLOW), duodenum, and small intestine after a liquid contrast substance (barium sulfate) is swallowed. In a small bowel follow-through, pictures are taken at increasing time intervals to follow the progress of barium through the small intestine. Identification of obstructions or ulcers is possible.

Urography (u-ROG-rah-fe) or **urogram** (UR-o-gram): X-ray recording of the kidney and urinary tract. If x-rays are taken after contrast medium is injected intravenously, the procedure is called *intravenous urography (descending* or *excretion urography)* or *intravenous pyelography (IVP).* If x-rays are taken after injection of contrast medium into the bladder through the urethra, the procedure is *retrograde urography* or *retrograde pyelography.* PYEL/O- means renal pelvis (the collecting chamber of the kidney).

NUCLEAR MEDICINE SCANS

In the following diagnostic tests, radioactive material *(radioisotope)* is injected intravenously or inhaled, and detected with a scanning device in the organ in which it accumulates. X-rays, ultrasound, or magnetic waves are not used.

Bone scan: A radioactive substance is injected intravenously, and its uptake in bones is detected with a scanning device. Tumors in bone can be detected by increased uptake of the radioactive material in the areas of the lesions.

Brain scan: A radioactive substance is injected intravenously. It collects in any lesion that disturbs the natural barrier that exists between blood vessels and normal brain tissue (blood-brain barrier), allowing the radioactive substance to enter the brain tissue. A scanning device detects the presence of the radioactive substance and thus can identify an area of tumor, abscess, or hematoma.

Gallium scan (GAL-le-um skan):   Radioactive gallium (gallium citrate) is injected into the bloodstream and is detected in the body with a scanning device that produces an image of the areas where gallium collects. The gallium collects in areas of certain tumors (Hodgkin disease) and in areas of infection.

MUGA scan (MUH-gah skan):   Test that uses radioactive technetium to measure cardiac output. Also called *technetium-99m ventriculography* or *multiple-gated acquisition* scan.

Positron emission tomography (POS-i-tron e-MISH-un to-MOG-rah-fe) or **PET scan:**   Radioactive substances (oxygen and glucose are used) that release radioactive particles called positrons are injected into the body and travel to specialized areas such as the brain and heart. Because of the way that the positrons are released, cross-sectional color pictures can be made showing the location of the radioactive substance. The most common use for PET scans is to detect tumors, which take up the radioactive substance (isotope) and appear as "hot spots" on the film.

Pulmonary perfusion scan (PUL-mo-ner-e per-FU-shun skan):   Radioactive particles are injected intravenously and travel rapidly to areas of the lung that are adequately filled with blood. Regions of obstructed blood flow caused by tumor, blood clot, swelling, and inflammation can be seen as nonradioactive areas on the scan.

Pulmonary ventilation scan (PUL-mo-ner-e ven-ti-LA-shun skan):   Radioactive gas is inhaled, and a special camera detects its presence in the lungs. The scan is used to detect lung segments that fail to fill with the radioactive gas. Lack of filling is usually due to diseases that obstruct the bronchial tubes and air sacs. This scan is also used in the evaluation of lung function before surgery.

Technetium-99m Sestamibi scan (tek-NE-she-um 99m ses-ta-MIH-be skan):   Technetium 99m Sestamibi is injected and taken up in areas of myocardial infarction (heart attack). This test can be used with an *exercise tolerance test (ETT-MIBI)* and is helpful in defining areas of poor blood flow to heart muscle.

Thallium-201 scintigraphy (THAL-e-um-201 SIN-tih-gra-fe): Thallium-201 is injected into a vein and images of blood flow through heart muscle are recorded. Cold spots correlate with areas of myocardial infarction. *Sestamibi scans (ETT-MIBI)* are also used to assess the status of blood flow through heart muscle during an exercise stress test.

Thyroid scan (THI-royd skan): A radioactive iodine chemical is injected intravenously and collects in the thyroid gland. A scanning device detects the radioactive substance in the gland, measuring it and producing an image of the gland. The increased or decreased activity of the gland is demonstrated by the gland's capacity to use the radioactive iodine. A thyroid scan evaluates the position, size, and functioning of the thyroid gland.

CLINICAL PROCEDURES

The following procedures are performed on patients to establish a correct diagnosis of an abnormal condition. In some instances, the procedure may also be used to treat the condition.

Abdominocentesis (ab-dom-in-o-sen-TE-sis): See PARACENTESIS.

Allergy test (AL-er-je test): A small quantity of various suspected allergic substances is applied to the skin and a reaction is noted.

Amniocentesis (am-ne-o-sen-TE-sis): Surgical puncture to remove fluid from the sac (amnion) that surrounds the fetus in the uterus. The fluid contains cells from the fetus that can be examined with a microscope for chromosomal analysis. Levels of chemicals in amniotic fluid also can detect defects in the fetus.

Arthrocentesis (ar-thro-sen-TE-sis): Surgical puncture to remove fluid from a joint.

Aspiration (as-peh-RA-shun): Withdrawal of fluid by suction through a needle or tube. The term *aspiration pneumonia* refers to an infection caused by inhalation into the lungs of food or an object.

Audiometry (aw-de-OM-eh-tre): Test using sound waves of various frequencies (e.g., 500 Hz) up to 8000 Hz, which quantifies the extent and type of hearing loss. An *audiogram* is the record produced by this test.

Auscultation (aw-skul-TA-shun): Process of listening for sounds produced within the body. This is most often performed with the aid of a stethoscope to determine the condition of the chest or abdominal organs or to detect the fetal heartbeat.

Biopsy (BI-op-se): Removal of a piece of tissue from the body and subsequent examination of the tissue with a microscope. The procedure is performed with a surgical knife, by needle aspiration, or via endoscopic removal (using a special forceps-like instrument inserted through a hollow flexible tube.) An *excisional biopsy* means that the entire tissue to be examined is removed. An *incisional biopsy* is the removal of only a small amount of tissue, and a *needle biopsy* indicates that tissue is pierced with a hollow needle and fluid is withdrawn for microscopic examination.

Bone marrow biopsy (bon MAH-ro BI-op-se):   Removal of a small amount of bone marrow. The cells are then examined with a microscope. Often the hip bone (iliac crest) is used, and the biopsy is helpful in determining the number and type of blood cells in the bone marrow. Also called a bone marrow aspiration.

Bronchoscopy (brong-KOS-ko-pe):   Insertion of a flexible tube (endoscope) into the airway. The lining of the bronchial tubes can be seen, and tissue may be removed for biopsy. The tube is usually inserted through the mouth but can also be directly inserted into the airway during mediastinoscopy. Sedation is required for this procedure.

Chorionic villus sampling (kor-e-ON-ik VIL-us SAM-pling):   Removal and microscopic analysis of a small piece of placental tissue to detect fetal abnormalities.

Colonoscopy (ko-lon-OS-ko-pe):   Insertion of a flexible tube (endoscope) through the rectum and into and upward through the colon for visual examination. Biopsy samples may be taken and benign growths, such as polyps, removed through the endoscope. The removal of a polyp is a *polypectomy* (pol-eh-PEK-to-me).

Colposcopy (kol-POS-ko-pe):   Inspection of the cervix through the insertion of a special microscope into the vagina. The vaginal walls are held apart with a speculum so that the cervix (entrance to the uterus) can come into view.

Conization (ko-nih-ZA-shun):   Removal of a cone-shaped sample of uterine cervix tissue. This sample is then examined with a microscope for evidence of cancerous growth. The special shape of the tissue sample allows the pathologist to examine the transitional zone of the cervix, where cancers are most likely to develop.

Culdocentesis (kul-do-sen-TE-sis):   Insertion of a thin, hollow needle through the vagina into the cul-de-sac, the space between the rectum and the uterus. Fluid is withdrawn and analyzed for evidence of cancerous cells, infection, or blood cells.

Cystoscopy (sis-TOS-ko-pe):   Insertion of a thin tube or cystoscope (endoscope) into the urethra and then into the urinary bladder to visualize the bladder and remove stones. A biopsy of the urinary bladder can be performed through the cystoscope.

Digital rectal examination (DIG-ih-tal REK-tal eks-am-ih-NA-shun):   A physician inserts a gloved finger into the rectum to detect rectal cancer and as a primary method to detect prostate cancer. The abbreviation is *DRE*.

Dilation and curettage (di-LA-shun and kur-eh-TAJ):   A series of probes of increasing size is systematically inserted through the vagina into the opening of the cervix. The cervix is thus dilated (widened) so that a curette (spoon-shaped instrument) can be inserted to remove tissue from the lining of the uterus. The tissue is then examined with a microscope. The abbreviation for this procedure is *D&C*.

Electrocardiography (e-lek-tro-kar-de-OG-rah-fe):   Connection of electrodes (wires or "leads") to the body to record electric impulses from the heart. The *electrocardiogram* is the actual record produced; it is useful in discovering abnormalities in heart rhythms and diagnosing heart disorders. The abbreviation is *EKG* or *ECG*.

Electroencephalography (e-lek-tro-en-sef-ah-LOG-rah-fe):   Connection of electrodes (wires or "leads") to the scalp to record electricity coming from within the brain. The *electroencephalogram* is the actual record produced. It is useful in the diagnosis and monitoring of epilepsy and other brain lesions and in the investigation of neurological disorders. It is also used to evaluate patients in coma (brain inactivity) and in the study of sleep disorders. The abbreviation is *EEG*.

Electromyography (e-lek-tro-mi-OG-rah-fe):   Insertion of needle electrodes into muscle to record electrical activity. This procedure detects injuries and diseases that affect muscles and nerves. The abbreviation is *EMG*.

Endoscopy (en-DOS-ko-pe):   Insertion of a thin, tube-like instrument (endoscope) into an organ or cavity. The endoscope is placed through a natural opening (the mouth or anus) or into a surgical incision, such as through the abdominal wall. Endoscopes contain bundles of glass fibers that carry light (fiberoptic); some instruments are equipped with a small forceps-like device that withdraws a sample of tissue for microscopic study (biopsy). Examples of endoscopy are bronchoscopy, colonoscopy, esophagoscopy, gastroscopy, and laparoscopy.

Esophagogastroduodenoscopy (eh-SOF-ah-go-GAS-tro-du-o-den-NOS-ko-pe):   Insertion of an endoscope through the mouth into the esophagus, stomach, and first part of the small intestine. Also called *EGD*.

Esophagoscopy (eh-sof-ah-GOS-ko-pe):   Insertion of an endoscope through the mouth and throat into the esophagus. Visual examination of the esophagus to detect ulcers, tumors, or other lesions is thus possible.

Excisional biopsy (ek-SIZ-in-al BI-op-se):   See biopsy.

Exophthalmometry (eks-of-thal-MOM-eh-tre):   Measurement of the extent of protrusion of the eyeball in *exophthalmos*.

Frozen section (fro-zen SEK-shun):   Quick preparation of a biopsy sample for examination during an actual surgical procedure. Tissue is taken from the operating room to the pathology laboratory and frozen. It is then thinly sliced and immediately examined with a microscope to determine whether the sample is benign or malignant and to determine the status of margins.

Gastroscopy (gas-TROS-ko-pe):   Insertion of an endoscope through the esophagus into the stomach for visual examination and/or biopsy of the stomach. When the upper portion of the small intestine is also visualized, the procedure is called *EGD* or *esophagogastroduodenoscopy*.

Holter monitor (HOL-ter ECG MON-ih-ter):   Electrocardiographic record of heart activity over an extended period of time. The Holter monitor is worn by the patient as normal daily activities are performed. It detects and aids in the management of heart rhythm abnormalities. Also called *ambulatory electrocardiograph*.

Hysteroscopy (his-ter-OS-ko-pe):   Insertion of an endoscope into the uterus for visual examination.

Incisional biopsy (in-SIZ-in-al BI-op-se):   See biopsy.

Laparoscopy (lap-ah-ROS-ko-pe):   Insertion of an endoscope into the abdomen. After the patient receives a local anesthetic, a laparoscope is inserted through an incision in the abdominal wall. This procedure gives the physician a view of the abdominal cavity, the surface of the liver and spleen, and the pelvic region. Laparoscopy is used to remove organs (such as the gallbladder, appendix, ovary) and tumors and for fallopian tube ligation to prevent pregnancy.

Laryngoscopy (lah-rin-GOS-ko-pe):   Insertion of an endoscope into the airway to visually examine the voice box (larynx). A laryngoscope transmits a magnified image of the larynx through a system of lenses and mirrors. The procedure can reveal tumors and explain changes in the voice. Sputum samples and tissue biopsies are obtained by using brushes or forceps attached to the laryngoscope.

Mediastinoscopy (me-de-ah-sti-NOS-ko-pe):   Insertion of an endoscope into the mediastinum (space in the chest between the lungs and in front of the heart). A mediastinoscope is inserted through a small incision in the neck while the patient is under anesthesia. This procedure is used to biopsy lymph nodes and to examine other structures within the mediastinum.

Muscle biopsy (MUS-el BI-op-se):   A sample of muscle tissue is removed and analyzed microscopically.

Needle biopsy (NE-dl BI-op-se):   See BIOPSY.

Ophthalmoscopy (of-thal-MOS-ko-pe):   A physician uses an *ophthalmoscope* to look directly into the eye, evaluating the optic nerve, retina, and blood vessels in the back of the eye and the lens in the front of the eye for cataracts. In *fluorescein angiography*, a contrast is injected intravenously and movement of blood in the back of the eye is observed with ophthalmoscopy.

Otoscopy (o-TOS-ko-pe):   A physician uses an *otoscope* inserted into the ear canal to check for obstructions (e.g., wax), infection, fluid, and eardrum perforations or scarring.

Palpation (pal-PA-shun):   Examination by touch. This is a technique of manual physical examination by which a doctor feels underlying tissues and organs through the skin.

Pap smear (pap smer):   Insertion of a cotton swab or wooden spatula into the vagina to obtain a sample of cells from the outer surface of the cervix (neck of the uterus). The cells are then smeared on a glass slide, preserved, and sent to the laboratory for microscopic examination. This test for cervical cancer was developed and named after the late Dr. George Papanicolaou. Results are reported as a Grade I to IV (I = normal, II = inflammatory, III = suspicious of malignant disease, IV = malignant disease).

Paracentesis (pah-rah-sen-TE-sis):   Surgical puncture of the membrane surrounding the abdomen (peritoneum) to remove fluid from the abdominal cavity. Fluid is drained for analysis and to prevent its accumulation in the abdomen. Also known as *abdominocentesis*.

Pelvic exam (PEL-vik ek-ZAM):   Physician examines female sex organs and checks the uterus and ovaries for enlargement, cysts, tumors, or abnormal bleeding. This is also known as an "internal exam."

Percussion (per-KUSH-un):   The technique of striking a part of the body with short, sharp taps of the fingers to determine the size, density, and position of the underlying parts by the sound obtained. Percussion is commonly used on the abdomen to examine the liver.

Proctosigmoidoscopy (prok-to-sig-moy-DOS-ko-pe):   Insertion of an endoscope through the anus to examine the first 10 to 12 inches of the rectum and colon. When the sigmoid colon is visualized with a longer endoscope, the procedure is called *sigmoidoscopy*. The procedure detects polyps, malignant tumors, and sources of bleeding.

Pulmonary function test (PUL-mo-ner-e FUNG-shun test):   Measurement of the air taken into and exhaled from the lungs by means of an instrument called a *spirometer*. The test may be abnormal in patients with asthma, chronic bronchitis, emphysema, and occupational exposures to asbestos, chemicals, and dusts.

Sigmoidoscopy (sig-moy-DOS-ko-pe):   See PROCTOSIGMOIDOSCOPY.

Stool culture (stool KUL-chur):   Feces (stools) placed in a growth medium (culture) are analyzed microscopically for evidence of microorganisms (bacteria).

Stress test (stress test):   An electrocardiogram taken during exercise. It may reveal hidden heart disease or confirm the cause of cardiac symptoms.

Thoracentesis (thor-ah-sen-TE-sis):   Insertion of a needle into the chest to remove fluid from the space surrounding the lungs (pleural cavity). After injection of a local anesthetic, a hollow needle is placed through the skin and muscles of the back and into the space between the lungs and chest wall. Fluid is then withdrawn by applying suction. Excess fluid *(pleural effusion)* may be a sign of infection or malignant disease. This procedure is used to diagnose conditions, to drain a pleural effusion, or to reexpand a collapsed lung *(atelectasis)*.

Thoracoscopy (tho-ra-KOS-ko-pe):   Insertion of an endoscope through an incision in the chest to visually examine the surface of the lungs. VATS is *video-assisted thoracoscopy (thorascopy)*.

Tuning fork tests (TOO-ning fork tests):   Tests of hearing using a vibrating tuning fork of known frequency as a source of sound.

LABORATORY TESTS

The following laboratory tests are performed on samples of a patient's blood, *plasma* (fluid portion of the blood), *serum* (plasma minus clotting proteins and produced after blood has clotted), urine, feces, *sputum* (mucus coughed up from the lungs), *cerebrospinal fluid* (fluid within the spaces around the spinal cord and brain), and skin.

Acid phosphatase (AH-sid FOS-fah-tas):   Measurement of the amount of an enzyme called *acid phosphatase* in serum. Enzyme levels are elevated in metastatic prostate cancer. Moderate elevations of this enzyme occur in diseases of bone and when breast cancer cells invade bone tissue.

Albumin (al-BU-min):   Measurement of the amount of albumin (protein) in both the serum and the urine. A decrease of albumin in serum indicates disease of the kidneys, malnutrition, or liver disease or may occur in extensive loss of protein in the gut or from the skin, as in a burn. The presence of albumin in the urine *(albuminuria)* indicates malfunction of the kidney.

Alkaline phosphatase (AL-kah-lin FOS-fah-tas):   Measurement of the amount of *alkaline phosphatase* (an enzyme found on cell membranes) in serum. Levels are elevated in liver diseases (such as hepatitis and hepatoma) and in bone disease and bone cancer. The laboratory symbol is *alk phos*.

Alpha-fetoprotein (al-fa-fe-to-PRO-teen):   Determination of the presence of a protein called alpha-globulin in serum. The protein is normally present in the serum of the fetus, infant, and pregnant woman. In fetuses with abnormalities of the brain and spinal cord, the protein leaks into the amniotic fluid surrounding the fetus and is an indicator of spinal tube defect (spina bifida) or anencephaly (lack of brain development). High levels are found in patients with cancer of the liver and other malignant diseases (testicular and ovarian cancers). Serum levels monitor the effectiveness of cancer treatment. Elevated levels are also seen in benign liver disease such as cirrhosis and viral hepatitis. The laboratory symbol is *AFP*.

ALT: Measurement of the amount of the enzyme called *alanine transaminase* in serum. The enzyme is normally present in blood but accumulates in blood with damage to liver cells. Also called *SGPT*.

ANA: See ANTINUCLEAR ANTIBODY TEST.

Antinuclear antibody test (an-tih-NU-kle-ar AN-tih-bod-e test):   A sample of plasma is tested for the presence of antibodies that are found in patients with systemic lupus erythematosus. Laboratory symbol is *ANA*.

AST: Measurement of the enzyme *aspartate transaminase* in serum. The enzyme is normally present in blood but accumulates when there is damage to the heart or to liver cells. Also called *SGOT*.

Bacterial and fungal tests (bak-TER-e-al and FUNG-al tests):   Samples from skin lesions are analyzed microscopically to diagnose bacterial or fungal conditions.

Bence Jones protein (BENS jonz PRO-ten):   Measurement of the presence of the Bence Jones protein in serum or urine. Bence Jones protein is a fragment of a normal serum protein, an immunoglobulin, produced by cancerous bone marrow cells (myeloma cells). Normally it is not found in either blood or urine, but in *multiple myeloma* (a malignant condition of bone marrow), high levels of Bence Jones protein are detected in urine and serum.

Bilirubin (bil-ih-RU-bin):   Measurement of the amount of bilirubin, an orange-brown pigment, in serum and urine. Bilirubin is derived from hemoglobin, the oxygen-carrying protein in red blood cells. Its presence in high concentration in serum and urine causes *jaundice* (yellow coloration of the skin) and may indicate disease of the liver, obstruction of bile ducts, or a type of anemia that leads to excessive destruction of red blood cells.

Blood chemistry profile: A comprehensive blood test that is a biochemical examination of various substances in the blood using a computerized laboratory analyzer. Tests include calcium (bones), phosphorus (bones), urea (kidney), creatinine (kidney), bilirubin (liver), AST or SGOT (liver and heart muscle) and ALT or SGPT (liver), alkaline phosphatase (liver and bone), globulin (liver and immune disorders), and albumin (liver and kidney). Also called SMA or sequential multiple analysis. SMA-6, SMA-12, and SMA-18 indicate the number of blood elements tested.

Blood culture (blud KUL-chur): Test to determine whether infection is present in the bloodstream. A sample of blood is added to a special medium (food) that promotes the growth of microorganisms. The medium is then examined by a medical technologist for evidence of bacteria or other microbes.

Blood urea nitrogen (blud u-RE-ah NI-tro-jen): Measurement of the amount of urea (nitrogen-containing waste material) in serum. A high level of serum urea indicates poor kidney function because it is the kidney's job to remove urea from the bloodstream and filter it into urine. The laboratory symbol is *BUN*.

CA-125: Protein released into the bloodstream by ovarian cancer cells. Measurement of CA-125 determines response to treatment.

Calcium (KAL-se-um): Measurement of the amount of calcium in serum, plasma, or whole blood. Low blood levels are associated with abnormal functioning of nerves and muscles, and high blood levels indicate loss of calcium from bones, excessive intake of calcium, disease of the parathyroid glands, or cancer. The laboratory symbol is *Ca*.

Carbon dioxide (KAR-bon di-OK-side): Blood test to measure the gas produced in tissues and eliminated by the lungs. Abnormal levels may reflect lung disorders. The laboratory symbol is CO_2.

Carcinoembryonic antigen (kar-sih-no-em-bree-ON-ik AN-ti-jen): A plasma test for a protein normally found in the blood of human fetuses and produced in healthy adults only in a very small amount, if at all. High levels of this antigen may be a sign of one of a variety of cancers, especially colon or pancreatic cancer. This test monitors the response of patients to cancer treatment. The laboratory abbreviation is *CEA*.

Cerebrospinal fluid (seh-re-bro-SPI-nal FLU-id): Measurement of cerebrospinal fluid for protein, sugar, and blood cells. The fluid is also cultured to detect microorganisms. Chemical tests are performed on specimens of the fluid removed by *lumbar puncture*. Abnormal conditions such as meningitis, brain tumor, and encephalitis are detected. The laboratory abbreviation is *CSF*.

Cholesterol (ko-LES-ter-ol): Measurement of the amount of cholesterol (substance found in animal fats and oils, egg yolks, and milk) in serum or plasma. Normal values vary for age and diet; levels above 200 mg/dl indicate a need for further testing and efforts to reduce cholesterol level because high levels are associated with hardening of arteries and heart disease. Blood is also tested for the presence of a lipoprotein substance that is a combination of cholesterol and protein. High levels (optimum level is 60 to 100 mg/dl) of *HDL* (high-density lipoprotein) cholesterol in the blood are beneficial because HDL cholesterol promotes the removal and excretion of excess cholesterol from the body, whereas high levels of low-density lipoprotein *(LDL)* are associated with the development of atherosclerosis (optimum level is 100 mg/dl or less).

Complete blood count: Determinations of the numbers of leukocytes (white blood cells), erythrocytes (red blood cells), and platelets (clotting cells). The CBC is useful in diagnosis of anemia, infection, and blood cell disorders, such as leukemia.

Creatine kinase (KRE-ah-tin KI-nas):   Measurement of levels of creatine kinase, a blood enzyme. Creatine kinase is normally found in heart muscle, brain tissue, and skeletal muscle. The presence of one form *(isoenzyme)* of creatine kinase (either CK-MB or CK2) in the blood is strongly indicative of recent myocardial infarction (heart attack) because the enzyme is released from heart muscle when the muscle is damaged or dying.

Creatinine (kre-AT-tih-nin):   Measurement of the amount of creatinine, a nitrogen-containing waste material, in serum or plasma. It is the most reliable test for kidney function. Because creatinine is normally produced as a protein breakdown product in muscle and is excreted by the kidney in urine, an elevation in the creatinine level in the blood indicates a disturbance of kidney function. Elevations are also seen in high-protein diets and dehydration.

Creatinine clearance (kre-AT-tih-nin KLER-ans):   Measurement of the rate at which creatinine is cleared (filtered) by the kidneys from the blood. A low creatinine clearance indicates that the kidneys are not functioning effectively to clear creatinine from the bloodstream and filter it into urine.

Culture (KUL-chur):   Identification of microorganisms in a special laboratory medium (fluid, solid, or semisolid material). In *sensitivity* tests, culture plates containing a specific microorganism are prepared and antibiotic-containing disks are applied to the culture surface. After overnight incubation, the area surrounding the disk (where growth was inhibited) is measured to determine whether the antibiotic is effective against the specific organism.

Differential (di-fer-EN-shul):   See WHITE BLOOD CELL COUNT.

Electrolytes (e-LEK-tro-litz):   Determination of the concentration of *electrolytes* (chemical substances capable of conducting an electric current) in serum or whole blood. When dissolved in water, electrolytes break apart into charged particles *(ions)*. The positively charged electrolytes are *sodium* (Na^+), *potassium* (K^+), *calcium* (Ca^{++}), and *magnesium* (Mg^{++}). The negatively charged electrolytes are *chloride* (Cl^-) and *bicarbonate* (HCO_3^-). These charged particles should be present at all times for proper functioning of cells. An electrolyte imbalance occurs when serum concentration is either too high or too low. Calcium balance can affect the bones, kidneys, gastrointestinal tract, and neuromuscular activity, and sodium balance affects blood pressure, nerve functioning, and fluid levels surrounding cells. Potassium balance affects heart and muscular activity.

Electrophoresis: See SERUM PROTEIN ELECTROPHORESIS.

ELISA (eh-LI-zah):   A laboratory assay (test) for the presence of antibodies to the AIDS virus. If a patient has positive results, it is likely that his/her blood contains the AIDS virus (HIV or human immunodeficiency virus). The presence of the virus stimulates white blood cells to make antibodies that are detected by the ELISA assay. This is the first test done to detect AIDS infection and is followed by a Western blot test to confirm the results. ELISA is an acronym for *enzyme-linked immunosorbent assay*.

Erythrocyte sedimentation rate (eh-RITH-ro-sit sed-ih-men-TA-shun rat): Measurement of the rate at which red blood cells (erythrocytes) in well-mixed venous blood settle to the bottom (sediment) of a test tube. If the rate of sedimentation is markedly slow (elevated sed rate), it may indicate inflammatory conditions, such as rheumatoid arthritis, or conditions that produce excessive proteins in the blood. Laboratory symbols are *ESR* and *sed rate.*

Estradiol (es-tra-DI-ol):   Test for the concentration of estradiol, which is a form of estrogen (female hormone) in serum, plasma, or urine.

Estrogen receptor assay (ES-tro-jen re-SEP-tor AS-a):   Test, performed at the time of a biopsy, to determine whether a sample of tumor contains an estrogen receptor protein. The protein, if present on breast cancer cells, combines with estrogen, allowing estrogen to promote the growth of the tumor. Thus if an estrogen receptor assay test is positive (the protein is present), then treatment with an antiestrogen drug would retard tumor growth. If the assay is negative (the protein is not present), then the tumor would not be affected by antiestrogen drug treatment.

Globulin (GLOB-u-lin):   Measurement (in serum) of proteins that bind to and destroy foreign substances (antigens). Globulins are made by cells of the immune system. *Gamma globulin* is one type of globulin that contains antibodies to fight disease.

Glucose (GLU-kos):   Measurement of the amount of glucose (sugar) in serum and plasma. High levels of glucose *(hyperglycemia)* indicate diseases such as diabetes mellitus and hyperthyroidism. Glucose is also measured in urine, and its presence indicates diabetes mellitus. *Fasting blood sugar test* is measurement of blood sugar after a patient has fasted.

Glucose tolerance test (GLU-kos TOL-er-ans test):   Test to determine how the body uses glucose. In the first part of this test, blood and urine samples are taken after the patient has fasted. Then a solution of glucose is given by mouth. A half hour after the glucose is taken, blood and urine samples are obtained again and are collected every hour for 4 to 5 hours. This test can indicate abnormal conditions such as diabetes mellitus, hypoglycemia, and liver or adrenal gland dysfunction.

Hematocrit (he-MAT-o-krit):   Measurement of the percentage blood volume occupied by red blood cells. The normal range is 40% to 50% in males and 37% to 47% in females. A low hematocrit indicates anemia. The laboratory symbol is *Hct.*

Hemoccult test (he-mo-KULT test):   Examination of small sample of stool for otherwise inapparent occult (hidden) traces of blood. The sample is placed on the surface of a collection kit and reacts with a chemical (e.g., guaiac). A positive result may indicate bleeding from polyps, ulcers, or malignant tumors. This is an important screening test for colon cancer. Also called a STOOL GUAIAC TEST.

Hemoglobin assay (HE-mo-glo-bin AS-a):   Measurement of the concentration of hemoglobin in blood. The normal blood hemoglobin ranges are 13.5 to 18.0 gm/dl in adult males and 12.0 to 16.0 gm/dl in adult females. The laboratory symbol is *Hgb.*

Human chorionic gonadotropin (HU-man kor-e-ON-ik go-nad-o-TRO-pin): Measurement of the concentration of human chorionic gonadotropin (a hormone secreted by cells of the fetal placenta) in urine. It is detected in urine within days after fertilization of egg and sperm cells and provides the basis of the most commonly used pregnancy test. The laboratory symbol is *hCG*.

Immunoassay (im-u-no-AS-a):   A method of testing blood and urine for the concentration of various chemicals, such as hormones, drugs, or proteins. The technique makes use of the immunological reaction between antigens and antibodies. An *assay* is a determination of the amount of any particular substance in fluid or tissue.

Immunohistochemistry (im-u-no-his-to-KEM-is-tre):   An antibody tagged with a radioactive or fluorescent label is spread over a tissue biopsy and used to detect the presence of an antigen (protein) produced by the tissue or infection.

Lipid tests (LIP-id tests):   Lipids are fatty substances such as cholesterol and triglycerides. See CHOLESTEROL and TRIGLYCERIDES.

Lipoprotein tests (li-po-PRO-teen tests):   See CHOLESTEROL.

Liver function tests (LIV-er FUNG-shun tests):   See ALKALINE PHOSPHATASE, BILIRUBIN, ALT, and AST.

Occult blood test: See HEMOCCULT TEST.

PKU test: Test that determines whether the urine of a newborn baby contains substances called *phenylketones*. If so, the condition is called *phenylketonuria (PKU)*. Phenylketonuria occurs in infants born lacking a specific enzyme. If the enzyme is missing, high levels of *phenylalanine* (an amino acid) accumulate in the blood, affecting the infant's brain and causing mental retardation. This situation is prevented by placing the infant on a special diet that prevents accumulation of phenylalanine in the bloodstream.

Platelet count (PLAT-let kownt):   Determination of the number of clotting cells (platelets) in a sample of blood.

Potassium (po-TAHS-e-um):   Measurement of the concentration of potassium in serum. Potassium combines with other minerals (such as calcium) and is an important chemical for proper functioning of muscles, especially the heart muscle. The laboratory symbol is K^+. See also ELECTROLYTES.

Pregnancy test (PREG-nan-se test):   Measurement in blood or urine of *human chorionic gonadotropin* (hCG), a hormone secreted by the placenta early in pregnancy.

Progesterone receptor assay (pro-JES-teh-rone re-SEP-tor AS-a):   Test to determines whether a sample of tumor contains a progesterone receptor protein. A positive test identifies that a breast cancer tumor would be responsive to antihormone therapy.

Prostate-specific antigen (PROS-tat spe-SI-fic AN-ti-jen):   Blood test that measures the amount of an antigen elevated in all patients with prostatic cancer and in some with an inflamed prostate gland. The laboratory symbol is *PSA*.

Protein electrophoresis: See SERUM PROTEIN ELECTROPHORESIS.

Prothrombin time (pro-THROM-bin tim):   Measurement of the activity of factors in the blood that participate in clotting. Deficiency of any of these factors can lead to a prolonged prothrombin time and difficulty in blood clotting. The test is important as a monitor for patients taking anticoagulants, substances that block the activity of blood clotting factors and increase the risk of bleeding.

PSA: See PROSTATE-SPECIFIC ANTIGEN.

Red blood cell count: Test in which the number of erythrocytes in a sample of blood is counted. A low red blood cell count may indicate anemia. A high count can indicate *polycythemia vera.*

Rheumatoid factor (ROO-mah-toyd FAK-tor):   Detection of the abnormal protein *rheumatoid factor* in the serum. It is found in patients with rheumatoid arthritis.

Semen analysis (SE-men ah-NAL-ih-sis):   Microscopic examination of sperm cells to detect viability and motility of sperm cells.

Serum enzyme tests (SE-rum EN-zim tests):   Measurements of enzymes released into the bloodstream after a heart attack. Examples are creatine kinase (CK) and troponin I and troponin T.

Serum and urine tests (SE-rum and UR-in tests):   Measurements of hormones, electrolytes, and glucose among other substances as indicators of endocrine and other body functions.

Serum protein electrophoresis (SE-rum PRO-teen e-lek-tro-for-E-sis):   A procedure that separates proteins with an electric current. The material tested, such as serum, containing various proteins, is placed on paper or gel or in liquid, and under the influence of an electric current, the proteins separate (-PHORESIS means separation) so that they can be identified and measured. The procedure is also known as *protein electrophoresis.*

SGOT: See AST.

SGPT: See ALT.

Skin tests: Tests in which substances are applied to the skin or injected under the skin and the reaction of immune cells in the skin is observed. These tests detect a person's sensitivity to substances such as dust or pollen. They can also indicate whether a person has been exposed to the bacteria that cause tuberculosis or diphtheria.

Slit-lamp microscopy (slit-lamp mi-KROS-ko-pe):   Microscopic examination of anterior eye structures.

SMA: See BLOOD CHEMISTRY PROFILE.

Sodium: See ELECTROLYTES.

Sputum test (SPU-tum test):   Examination of mucus coughed up from a patient's lungs to detect tumor or infection. The sputum is examined microscopically and chemically and is cultured for the presence of microorganisms.

Stool guaiac test (stool GWI-ak test):   See HEMOCCULT TEST.

Thyroid function tests (THI-royd FUNG-shun tests):   Tests that measure the levels of thyroid hormones, such as *thyroxine* (T_4) and *triiodothyronine* (T_3), in serum. *Thyroid-stimulating hormone (TSH),* which is produced by the pituitary gland and stimulates the release of T_4 and T_3 from the thyroid gland, is also measured in serum. These tests diagnose hypothyroidism and hyperthyroidism and are helpful in monitoring response to thyroid treatment.

Triglyceride (tri-GLIS-er-ide):   Determination of the amount of triglycerides (simple fats) in the serum. Elevated triglyceride levels (normal is 200 mg to 300 mg/dL), are considered an important risk factor for the development of heart disease.

Troponin (tro-PO-nin):   Measurement of levels of proteins troponin I and troponin T in the bloodstream after myocardial injury (heart attack).

Uric acid (UR-ik AS-id):   Measurement of the amount of uric acid (a nitrogen-containing waste material) in the serum and urine. High serum levels indicate a type of arthritis called *gout.* In gout, uric acid accumulates as crystals in joints and in tissues. High levels of uric acid may also cause kidney stones.

Urinalysis (u-rih-NAL-ih-sis):   Examination of urine as an aid in the diagnosis of disease. Routine urinalysis involves the observation of unusual color or odor; determination of specific gravity (amount of materials dissolved in urine); chemical tests (for protein, sugar, acetone); and microscopic examination for bacteria, blood cells, and sediment. Urinalysis is used to detect abnormal functioning of the kidneys and bladder, infections, abnormal growths, and diabetes mellitus. The laboratory symbol is *UA.*

Western blot (WES-tern blot):   Test used to detect infection by *HIV* (AIDS virus). It is more specific than the ELISA. A patient's serum is mixed with purified proteins from HIV, and the reaction is examined. If the patient has made antibodies to HIV, those antibodies react with the purified HIV proteins and the test is positive.

White blood cell (WBC) count: Determination of the number of leukocytes in the blood. Higher than normal counts can indicate the presence of infection or leukemia. A *differential* is the percentages of different types of white blood cells (neutrophils, eosinophils, basophils, lymphocytes, and monocytes) in a sample of blood. It gives more specific information about leukocytes and aids in the diagnosis of infection, allergic diseases, disorders of the immune system, and various forms of leukemia.

Appendix III

Abbreviations, Acronyms, and Symbols

ABBREVIATIONS

𝒜

AB	abortion
Ab	antibody
ABC	aspiration, biopsy, cytology
abd	abdomen
a.c., ac	before meals *(ante cibum)*
ACE	angiotensin converting enzyme (ACE inhibitors treat hypertension)
ACL	anterior cruciate ligament (of knee)
ACS	acute coronary syndromes (myocardial infarction and unstable angina)
ACTH	adrenocorticotropic hormone (secreted by the pituitary gland)
ADD	attention deficit disorder
ADH	antidiuretic hormone (secreted by the pituitary gland)
ADHD	attention deficit hyperactivity disorder
ad lib	freely as desired *(ad libitum)*
AIDS	acquired immunodeficiency syndrome
alb	albumin (protein)
ALL	acute lymphocytic leukemia
alk phos	alkaline phosphatase (enzyme elevated in liver disease)
ALS	amyotrophic lateral sclerosis (Lou Gehrig disease)
ALT	alanine transaminase (enzyme elevated in liver disease); SGPT
AML	acute myelocytic (myelogenous) leukemia
AP or A/P	anteroposterior (front to back)
A&P	auscultation and percussion
aq	water *(aqua)*
ASD	atrial septal defect
ASHD	arteriosclerotic heart disease
AST	aspartate transaminase (elevated in liver and heart disease); SGOT
AV	arteriovenous; atrioventricular
A&W	alive and well

ℬ

BaE (BE)	barium enema
B cells	white blood cells (lymphocytes) produced in bone marrow
b.i.d., bid	twice a day *(bis in die)*
BM	bowel movement; bone marrow
BMT	bone marrow transplant
BP, B/P	blood pressure

BPH	benign prostatic hypertrophy (hyperplasia)
Bronch	bronchoscopy
bs	blood sugar; bowel sounds; breath sounds
BSE	breast self-examination
BSO	bilateral salpingo-oophorectomy
BUN	blood urea nitrogen (test of kidney function)
BW	birth weight
Bx, bx	biopsy

C

c̄	with *(cum)*
C1, C2	first, second cervical vertebra
CA	cancer; carcinoma; cardiac arrest; chronological age
Ca	calcium
CABG	coronary artery bypass graft
CAD	coronary artery disease
CAPD	continuous ambulatory peritoneal dialysis
cap	capsule
cath	catheter; catheterization
CBC	complete blood count
CC	chief complaint
CCU	coronary care unit; critical care unit
CF	cystic fibrosis
Chemo	chemotherapy
CHF	congestive heart failure
Chol	cholesterol
CIN	cervical intraepithelial neoplasia
CIS	carcinoma *in situ*
CKD	chronic kidney disease
cm	centimeter (1/100 meter)
CML	chronic myelocytic (myelogenous) leukemia
CNS	central nervous system
c/o	complains of
CO₂	carbon dioxide
COPD	chronic obstructive pulmonary disease
CP	cerebral palsy; chest pain
CPD	cephalopelvic disproportion
CPR	cardiopulmonary resuscitation
C&S, C+S	culture and sensitivity
C-section, CS	cesarean section
CSF	cerebrospinal fluid
CT	computed tomography (see CT scan)
CT (CAT) scan	computed axial tomography (x-ray images in cross-sectional view)
CVA	cerebrovascular accident (stroke)

c/w	consistent with
CXR, CX	chest x-ray
cysto	cystoscopy

𝒟

D&C	dilation and curettage (of the uterine lining)
DES	diethylstilbestrol (estrogen causing defects in children whose mothers took the drug during pregnancy)
DIC	disseminated intravascular coagulation
diff	differential (percentages of types of white blood cells)
DKA	diabetic ketoacidosis
DM	diabetes mellitus
DNA	deoxyribonucleic acid
DOB	date of birth
DOE	dyspnea on exertion
DRE	digital rectal exam
DT	delirium tremens (caused by alcohol withdrawal)
DTR	deep tendon reflex
DVT	deep vein thrombosis
Dx	diagnosis

ℰ

EBV	Epstein-Barr virus (cause of mononucleosis)
ECC	emergency cardiac care
ECG (EKG)	electrocardiogram
Echo	echocardiogram
ECMO	extracorporeal membrane oxygenator
ECT	electroconvulsive therapy
ED	emergency department
EDC	estimated date of confinement
EEG	electroencephalogram
EENT	eyes, ears, nose, and throat
EGD	esophagogastroduodenoscopy
ELISA	enzyme-linked immunosorbent assay (AIDS test)
EMG	electromyogram
ENT	ears, nose, throat
Eos	eosinophil (type of white blood cell)
ER	emergency room; estrogen receptor
ERCP	endoscopic retrograde cholangiopancreatography
ESR	erythrocyte sedimentation rate; see sed rate
ESRD	end-stage renal disease
ESWL	extracorporeal shockwave lithotripsy
ETOH	ethyl alcohol (ethanol)
ETT	exercise tolerance test; endotracheal tube

$\mathcal{F}$

FBS	fasting blood sugar
FDA	Food and Drug Administration
Fe	iron
FEV	forced expiratory volume
FH	family history
FHR	fetal heart rate
FSH	follicle-stimulating hormone (secreted by the pituitary gland)
F/U, f/u	follow-up
FUO	fever of unknown (undetermined) origin
Fx	fracture

$\mathcal{G}$

g (gm)	gram
Ga	gallium (element used in nuclear medicine diagnostic tests)
GB	gallbladder
GC	gonococcus (bacterial cause of gonorrhea)
Gd	gadolinium (widely used MRI contrast agent)
GERD	gastroesophageal reflux disease
GH	growth hormone (secreted by the pituitary gland)
GI	gastrointestinal
Grav. 1, 2, 3	first, second, third pregnancy
gt, gtt	drop, drops
GTT	glucose tolerance test
GU	genitourinary
GVHD	graft versus host disease
Gyn	gynecology

$\mathcal{H}$

H	hydrogen
h, hr	hour
HBV	hepatitis B virus
HCG, hCG	human chorionic gonadotropin (secreted during pregnancy)
Hct	hematocrit
HCV	hepatitis C virus
HD	hemodialysis (artificial kidney machine)
HDL	high-density lipoproteins (associated with decreased incidence of coronary artery disease)
HEENT	head, ears, eyes, nose, and throat
Hg	mercury
Hgb	hemoglobin
HIPAA	Health Insurance Portability and Accountability Act (of 1996)
HIV	human immunodeficiency virus
h/o	history of

H₂O	water
H&P	history and physical
HPV	human papilloma virus
HRT	hormone replacement therapy
HSG	hysterosalpingography
HSV-1, 2	herpes simplex virus type 1, 2
HTN	hypertension (high blood pressure)
Hx	history

I

I	iodine
I&D	incision and drainage
IBD	inflammatory bowel disease (ulcerative colitis and Crohn disease)
IBS	irritable bowel syndrome (unknown etiology)
ICU	intensive care unit
I&D	incision & drainage
IM	intramuscular; infectious mononucleosis
INH	isoniazid (drug to treat tuberculosis)
I&O	intake and output (measurement of patient's fluids)
IOL	intraocular lens (implant)
IUD	intrauterine device (contraceptive)
IV	intravenous
IVP	intravenous pyelogram

K

K	potassium
kg	kilogram (1000 grams)
KS	Kaposi sarcoma (malignant disease associated with AIDS)
KUB	kidneys, ureters, bladder (x-ray image)

L

L, l	left; liter; lower
L1, L2	first, second lumbar vertebra
LA	left atrium
lat	lateral
LBP	low back pain; low blood pressure
LDH	lactate dehydrogenase (elevations associated with heart attacks)
LDL	low-density lipoproteins (high levels associated with heart disease)
LE	lupus erythematosus
LEEP	loop electrocautery excision procedure
LES	lower esophageal sphincter
LFT	liver function test

LLQ	left lower quadrant (of the abdomen)
LMP	last menstrual period
LP	lumbar puncture
LPN	licensed practical nurse
LTB	laryngotracheal bronchitis (croup)
LUQ	left upper quadrant (of the abdomen)
LV	left ventricle
LVAD	left ventricular assist device (bridge to transplant)
L&W	living and well
lymphs	lymphocytes
lytes	electrolytes

M

m	meter; milli (one thousandth)
μ	micro (one millionth)
MAC	monitored anesthesia care
MCH	mean corpuscular hemoglobin (amount in each red blood cell)
MCHC	mean corpuscular hemoglobin concentration (amount per unit of blood)
MCV	mean corpuscular volume (size of individual red blood cell)
MD, M.D.	doctor of medicine; muscular dystrophy
mets	metastases
mg	milligram (1/1000 gram)
Mg	magnesium
MH	marital history; mental health
MI	myocardial infarction (heart attack)
ml	milliliter (1/1000 liter)
mm	millimeter (1/1000 meter)
mm Hg	millimeters of mercury (measurement of blood pressure)
mono	monocytes (type of white blood cell)
MRA	magnetic resonance angiography
MRI	magnetic resonance imaging
MS	mitral stenosis; multiple sclerosis; mental status
MSW	medical social worker
MVP	mitral valve prolapse
myop	myopia (near-sightedness)

N

N	nitrogen
Na	sodium
NB	newborn
NED	no evidence of disease
NG tube	nasogastric tube
NICU	neonatal intensive care unit

NKA	no known allergies
NPO	nothing by mouth *(nil per os)*
NSAID	nonsteroidal anti-inflammatory drug
NSR	normal sinus rhythm (of the heart)
NTP	normal temperature and pressure
N+V	nausea and vomiting

O

O$_2$	oxygen
OA	osteoarthritis
OB	obstetrics
OD, O.D.	right eye *(oculus dexter)*; doctor of optometry
OR	operating room
ORIF	open reduction, internal fixation (to set a broken bone)
ORTH, ortho.	orthopedics or orthopaedics
os	mouth
OS	left eye *(oculus sinister)*
OSA	obstructive sleep apnea
OU	each eye *(oculus uterque)*
OV	office visit

P

p̄	after; following
P	plan; posterior; pulse; phosphorus; pupil; pressure
PA	posteroanterior (back to front); pulmonary artery
PAC	premature atrial contraction
PaCO$_2$	arterial pressure of carbon dioxide in the blood; also written PCO$_2$
PACS	picture archival communications system
palp	palpable; palpation (examine by touch)
PaO$_2$	arterial pressure of oxygen in the blood
Pap smear	Papanicolaou smear (microscopic examination of cells from the cervix and vagina)
para	paracentesis (abdominocentesis)
Para 1,2,3	woman having produced one, two, three viable offspring; unipara, bipara, tripara
p.c., pc	after meals *(post cibum)*
PCI	percutaneous coronary interventions
PE	physical examination; pulmonary embolus
PEEP	positive end-expiratory pressure
per	by
PERRLA	pupils equal, round, and reactive to light and accommodation
PET	positron emission tomography
PE tube	pressure-equalizing tube (ventilating tube for the eardrum)
PFT	pulmonary function test

pH	hydrogen ion concentration (measurement of acidity or alkalinity of a solution)
PH	past history
PI	present illness
PID	pelvic inflammatory disease
PKU	phenylketonuria (test for lack of an enzyme in infants)
PM	afternoon *(post meridian)*; postmortem
PMH	past medical history
PND	paroxysmal nocturnal dyspnea; postnasal drip
p/o	postoperative
p.o., po	by mouth *(per os)*
polys	polymorphonuclear leukocytes (neutrophils)
poplit	popliteal (behind the knee)
post-op	after operation
PP	after meals *(postprandial)*; after birth *(postpartum)*
PPD	purified protein derivative (skin test for tuberculosis)
pre-op	before operation (preoperative)
prep	prepare for
p.r.n., prn	as needed *(pro re nata)*
procto	proctoscopy (visual examination of the anus and rectum)
pro time	prothrombin time (test of blood clotting)
PSA	prostate-specific antigen
pt	patient
PT	physical therapy; prothrombin time
PTA	prior to admission (to hospital)
PTCA	percutaneous transluminal coronary angioplasty (balloon angioplasty)
PTH	parathyroid hormone
PTR	patient to return
PTT	partial thromboplastin time (test of blood clotting)
PVC	premature ventricular contraction (abnormal heart rhythm)
PVD	peripheral vascular disease
PVT	paroxysmal ventricular tachycardia
PWB	partial weight bearing

Q

q	every *(quaque)*
q.h., qh	each hour *(quaque hora)*
q2h	each two hours *(quaque secunda hora)*
q.i.d., qid	four times a day *(quater in die)*
q.n.s., qns	quantity not sufficient *(quantum non suffict)*
q.s., qs	quantity sufficient *(quantum suffict)*
qt	quart

ℛ

R, r	right; respiration
RA	rheumatoid arthritis; right atrium
rad	radiation absorbed dose
RBC, rbc	red blood cell (count)
RIA	radioimmunoassay (minute quantities are measured)
RLQ	right lower quadrant (of the abdomen)
R/O, r/o	rule out
ROM	range of motion
ROS	review of systems
RP	retrograde pyelogram (urogram)
RR	recovery room; respiration rate
RRR	regular rate and rhythm (of the heart)
RT	radiation therapy; recreational therapy; radiologic technologist
RUQ	right upper quadrant (of the abdomen)
RV	right ventricle (of the heart)
Rx	treatment (recipe)

S

s̄	without *(sine)*
S1, S2	first, second sacral vertebra
S-A node	sinoatrial node (pacemaker of the heart)
SARS	severe acute respiratory syndrome
SBFT	small bowel follow-through (x-rays of the small intestine with contrast)
sed. rate	erythrocyte sedimentation rate (time it takes red blood cells to settle out of blood)
segs	segmented white blood cells (granulocytes)
SERM	selective estrogen receptor modulator (tamoxifen is an example)
s.gl.	without glasses
SGOT	see AST
SGPT	see ALT
SH	social history: serum hepatitis
sig	let it be labeled
SIDS	sudden infant death syndrome
SIRS	systemic inflammatory response syndrome (severe bacteremia)
SLE	systemic lupus erythematosus
SMA	sequential multiple analyzer (test of blood components)
SOAP	subjective (symptoms perceived by the patient) data, objective (exam findings) data, assessment (evaluation of condition), plan (goals for treatment)
SOB	shortness of breath
S/P, s/p	status post (previous disease condition)
SPECT	single photon emission computed tomography

sp.gr.	specific gravity
SSRI	selective serotonin reuptake inhibitor (antidepressant drug)
staph	staphylococci (bacteria)
STAT, stat	immediately *(statim)*
STI	sexually transmitted infection
strep	streptococci (bacteria)
Sx	symptoms; signs
sz	seizure

T

T	temperature; time
T1, T2	first, second thoracic vertebra
T$_3$	triiodothyronine (thyroid gland hormone)
T$_4$	thyroxine (thyroid gland hormone)
T&A	tonsillectomy and adenoidectomy
tab	tablet
TAB	therapeutic abortion
TAH-BSO	total abdominal hysterectomy–bilateral salpingo-oophorectomy
TB	tuberculosis
T cells	lymphocytes originating in the thymus gland
TEE	transesophageal echocardiogram
TIA	transient ischemic attack
TENS	transcutaneous electrical nerve stimulator
THR	total hip replacement
t.i.d., tid	three times a day
TLC	total lung capacity
TM	tympanic membrane
TNM	tumor, nodes, metastasis (staging system for cancer)
tomos	tomograms (x-ray images to show an organ in depth)
TPN	total parenteral nutrition
TPR	temperature, pulse, respiration
TRUS	transrectal ultrasound
TSH	thyroid-stimulating hormone (secreted by the pituitary gland)
TUIP	transurethral incision of the prostate gland
TUR, TURP	transurethral resection of the prostate gland
TVH	total vaginal hysterectomy
Tx	treatment

U

UA, U/A	urinalysis
UE	upper extremity
UGI	upper gastrointestinal
umb	navel (umbilical cord region)
ung	ointment
U/O	urine output

URI	upper respiratory infection
US, u/s	ultrasound
UTI	urinary tract infection
UV	ultraviolet

$\mathcal{V}$

VA	visual acuity
VC	vital capacity (of lungs)
VCUG	voiding cystourethrogram
VF	visual field; ventricular fibrillation
VS, V/S	vital signs
VSD	ventricular septal defect
VSS	vital signs stable
V tach, VT	ventricular tachycardia (abnormal heart rhythm)

$\mathcal{W}$

WBC, wbc	white blood cell; white blood count
W/C	wheelchair
wd	wound
WDWN	well developed, well nourished
WNL	within normal limits
WT, wt	weight
w/u	work-up

$\mathcal{X}$

XRT	radiation therapy

$\mathcal{Y}$

y/o, yr	year(s) old

ACRONYMS*

An acronym is the name for an abbreviation that forms a pronounceable word.

ACE (ace)	angiotensin-converting enzyme
AIDS (ades)	acquired immune deficiency syndrome
BUN (bun)	blood, urea, nitrogen
CABG (cabbage)	coronary artery bypass graft
CAT (cat)	computerized axial tomography
CPAP (seepap)	continuous positive airway pressure
ELISA (eliza)	enzyme-linked immunosorbent assay
GERD (gerd)	gastroesphageal reflux disease
HAART (hart)	highly active antiretroviral therapy
HIPAA (hipa)	Health Insurance Portability and Accountability Act of 1996
LASER (lazer)	light amplification by stimulated emission of radiation
LASIK (lasik)	laser *in situ* keratomileusis
LEEP (leep)	loop electrocautery excision procedure
MICU (micku)	medical intensive care unit
MODS (mods)	multiorgan dysfunction syndrome
MUGA (mugah)	multiple-gated acquisition (scan)
NSAID (insayd)	nonsteroidal antiinflammatory drug
NICU (nicku)	neonatal intensive care unit
PACS (packs)	picture archival communications system
PALS (pals)	pediatric advanced life support
PEEP (peep)	positive end expiratory pressure
PEG (peg)	percutaneous endoscopic gastrostomy
PERRLA (perlah)	pupils equal, round, reactive to light and accommodation
PET (pet)	positron emission tomography
PICU (picku)	pediatric intensive care unit
PIP (pip)	proximal interphalangeal joint
PIXELS (pixels)	picture elements
PUVA (poovah)	psoralen ultraviolet A
REM (rem)	rapid eye movement
SAD (sad)	seasonal affective disorder
SARS (sarz)	severe acute respiratory syndrome
SERM (serm)	selective estrogen receptor modulator
SIDS (sidz)	sudden infant death syndrome
SIRS (sirs)	systemic inflammatory response syndrome
SMAC (smak)	sequential multiple analyzer computer (blood testing)
SOAP (soap)	subjective, objective, assessment, plan
SPECT (spekt)	single-photon emission computed tomography
TENS (tenz)	transcutaneous electrical nerve stimulation
TRUS (truss)	transrectal ultrasound
TURP (turp)	transurethral resection of the prostate
VATS (vats)	video-assisted thoracoscopy
VOXEL (voxel)	volume element (of CT scan)

*Modified from Chabner D-E: *The Language of Medicine,* ed 7, Philadelphia, 2004, WB Saunders.

SYMBOLS*

=	equal
≠	unequal
+	positive
−	negative
↑	above, increase
↓	below, decrease
♀	female
♂	male
→	to (in the direction of)
1°	primary to
2°	secondary to
ʒ	dram
℥	ounce
%	percent
°	degree; hour
:	ratio; "is to"
±	plus or minus (either positive or negative)
′	foot
″	inch
∴	therefore
@	at, each
c̄	with
s̄	without
#	pound
≈	approximately, about
Δ	change
p	short arm of a chromosome
q	long arm of a chromosome

*Modified from Chabner D-E: *The Language of Medicine,* ed 7, Philadelphia, 2004, WB Saunders.

Glossary of
Medical Terms

Pronunciation of each term is given with its meaning. The syllable that gets the accent is in CAPITAL LETTERS. Terms in SMALL CAPITAL LETTERS are defined elsewhere in the glossary.

A

Abdomen (AB-do-men): Space below the chest that contains organs such as the stomach, liver, intestines, and gallbladder. Also called the abdominal cavity, the abdomen lies between the diaphragm and the pelvis.

Abdominal (ab-DOM-i-nal): Pertaining to the abdomen.

Abdominal cavity (ab-DOM-i-nal KAV-ih-te): See ABDOMEN.

Abnormal (ab-NOR-mal): Pertaining to being away (AB-) from the norm; irregular.

Acquired immunodeficiency syndrome (ah-KWI-erd im-u-no-deh-FISH-en-se SIN-drom) or **AIDS:** Suppression or deficiency of the immune response caused by exposure to the HUMAN IMMUNODEFICIENCY VIRUS (HIV).

Acromegaly (ak-ro-MEG-ah-le): Enlargement of extremities as a result of thickening of the bones and soft tissues; it is caused by excessive secretion of growth hormone from the pituitary gland (after completion of puberty).

Acute (ah-KUT): Sharp, sudden, and intense for a short period of time.

Adenectomy (ad-eh-NEK-to-me): The removal of a gland.

Adenitis (ad-en-NI-tis): Inflammation of a gland.

Adenocarcinoma (ah-deh-no-kar-sih-NO-mah): Cancerous tumor derived from glandular cells.

Adenoidectomy (ah-deh-noyd-EK-to-me): Removal of the adenoids.

Adenoids (AD-eh-noidz): Enlarged lymphatic tissue in the upper part of the throat near the nasal passageways.

Adenoma (ah-deh-NO-mah): Benign tumor of glandular cells.

Adenopathy (ah-deh-NOP-ah-the): Disease of glands. Often this term refers to enlargement of lymph nodes (which are not true glands, but collections of lymphatic tissue).

Adnexa uteri (ad-NEKS-ah U-ter-i): Accessory structures of the uterus (ovaries and fallopian tubes).

Adrenal cortex (ah-DRE-nal KOR-teks): Outermost part of the adrenal gland. The adrenal cortex secretes steroid hormones such as GLUCOCORTICOIDS (cortisone).

Adrenal glands (ah-DRE-nal glanz): Two endocrine glands, each above a kidney. The adrenal glands produce hormones such as adrenalin (epinephrine) and hydrocortisone (cortisol).

Adrenalectomy (ah-dre-nal-EK-to-me): Removal (excision) of adrenal glands.

Adrenaline (ah-DREN-eh-lin): Hormone secreted by the adrenal glands. It is released into the bloodstream in response to stress, such as from fear or physical injury. Also called EPINEPHRINE.

Adrenocorticotropic hormone (ah-dre-no-kor-tih-ko-TROP-ic HOR-mon): Hormone secreted by the pituitary gland. It stimulates the adrenal gland (cortex or outer region) to secrete the hormone cortisone. Also called ACTH.

Adrenopathy (ah-dre-NOP-a-the): Disease of ADRENAL GLANDS.

AIDS: See ACQUIRED IMMONODEFICIENCY SYNDROME.

Air sacs (ayr saks):   Thin-walled sacs within the lung. Inhaled oxygen passes into the blood from the sacs, and carbon dioxide passes out from the blood into the sacs to be exhaled.

Albuminuria (al-bu-men-U-re-ah):   Albumin (protein) in the urine; it indicates a malfunction of the kidney.

Alkaline phosphatase (AL-kah-line PHOS-phah-tase):   An enzyme present in blood and body tissues, such as bone and liver. Elevated in diseases such as those of bone and liver. Also called alk phos.

Allergist (AL-er-jist):   Medical doctor specializing in identifying and treating abnormal sensitivity to foreign substances such as pollen, dust, foods, and drugs.

Alopecia (ah-lo-PE-shah):   Loss of hair; baldness.

ALT: An enzyme normally found in blood and tissues, especially the liver. Also known as SGPT; elevated in liver disease.

Alveolar (al-VE-o-lar):   Pertaining to air sacs (alveoli) within the lungs.

Alveolus (al-ve-O-lus):   An air sac within the lung (pl. alveoli).

Alzheimer disease (ALTZ-hi-mer di-ZEZ):   Deterioration of mental capacity (irreversible dementia) marked by intellectual deterioration, disorganization of personality, and difficulties in carrying out tasks of daily living.

Amenorrhea (a-men-o-RE-ah):   Absence of menstrual periods.

Amniocentesis (am-ne-o-sen-TE-sis):   Surgical puncture to remove fluid from the amnion (sac surrounding the developing fetus).

Anal (A-nal):   Pertaining to the anus (opening of the rectum to the outside of the body).

Analgesic (an-al-JE-zik):   Medication that reduces or eliminates pain.

Analysis (ah-NAL-ih-sis):   Separating a substance into its component parts.

Anastomosis (ah-na-sto-MO-sis):   New surgical connection between two previously unconnected bowel parts, vessels, or ducts.

Androgen (AN-dro-jen):   Hormone that controls the development of masculine characteristics. An example is TESTOSTERONE.

Anemia (ah-NE-me-ah):   Deficiency of hemoglobin and/or numbers of red blood cells, which results in reduced oxygen to body cells. Literally, *anemia* means lacking (AN-) in blood (-EMIA).

Anemic (ah-NE-mik):   Pertaining to ANEMIA.

Anesthesiologist (an-es-the-ze-OL-o-jist):   Medical doctor specializing in administering agents capable of bringing about loss of sensation and consciousness.

Anesthesiology (an-es-the-ze-OL-o-je):   Study of how to administer agents capable of bringing about loss of sensation and consciousness.

Aneurysm (AN-u-rizm):   Localized widening of the wall of an artery, of a vein, or of the heart. From the Greek *aneurysma* meaning "widening."

Angina (an-JI-nah):   Sharp pain in the chest resulting from a decrease in blood supply to heart muscle. Also called angina pectoris (chest).

Angiography (an-je-OG-rah-fe):   X-ray recording of blood vessels after contrast is injected.

Angioplasty (AN-je-o-plas-te):   Surgical repair of a blood vessel. A tube (catheter) is placed in a clogged artery and a balloon at the end of the tube is inflated to flatten the clogged material against the wall of the artery. This enlarges the opening of the artery so that more blood can pass through. Also called balloon angioplasty.

Angiotensin (AN-je-o-TEN-sin):   Hormone that is a powerful vasoconstrictor and raises blood pressure.

Ankylosing spondylitis (ang-ki-LO-sing spon-dih-LI-tis):   Chronic inflammation of the vertebrae (backbones) with stiffening of spinal joints so that movement becomes increasingly painful.

Ankylosis (ang-ki-LO-sis):   Stiffening and immobility of a joint caused by injury, disease, or a surgical procedure.

Anomaly (an-NOM-ah-le):   Irregularity; a deviation from the normal. A congenital anomaly (irregularity) is present at birth.

Antenatal (AN-te NA-tal):   Before birth.

Antepartum (AN-te PAR-tum):   Before birth.

Anterior (an-TE-re-or):   Located in the front (of the body or of a structure).

Antiandrogen (an-tih-AN-dro-jen):   Substance that inhibits the effects of androgens (male hormones).

Antiarrhythmic (an-te-ah-RITH-mik):   Pertaining to a drug that works against or prevents abnormal heartbeats (arrhythmias).

Antibiotic (an-tih-bi-OT-ik):   Pertaining to a substance that works against germ or bacterial life.

Antibody (AN-tih-bod-e):   A substance that works against (ANTI-) germs ("bodies" of infection). Antibodies are produced by white blood cells when germs (antigens) enter the bloodstream.

Anticoagulant (an-tih-ko-AG-u-lant):   Drug that prevents clotting (coagulation). Anticoagulants are given when there is danger of clots forming in blood vessels.

Anticonvulsant (an-tih-kon-VULS-ent):   Drug that prevents or relieves convulsions (involuntary muscular contractions).

Antidepressant (an-tih-de-PRES-ent):   Drug used to prevent or treat depression.

Antidiabetic (an-tih-di-ah-BET-ik):   Drug that prevents or relieves symptoms of diabetes.

Antiestrogen (an-tih-ES-tro-jen):   Substance that inhibits the effects of estrogens (female hormones).

Antifungal (an-tih-FUNG-al):   Drug that destroys or inhibits the growth of fungi (organisms such as yeasts, molds, and mushrooms).

Antigen (AN-tih-jen):   Foreign protein (such as on a bacterium or virus) that stimulates white blood cells to make antibodies. Antigens are then destroyed by the antibodies.

Antihistamine (an-tih-HIS-tah-men):   Drug used to counteract the effects of histamine production in allergic reactions and colds.

Antihypertensive (an-ti-hi-per-TEN-siv):   Drug that reduces high blood pressure.

Antitubercular (an-tih-too-BER-ku-lar):   Agent or drug used to treat tuberculosis.

Antiviral (an-tih-VI-ral):   Agent that inhibits and prevents the growth and reproduction of viruses.

Anuria (an-U-re-ah):   Lack of urine formation by the kidney.

Anus (A-nus):   Opening of the rectum to the surface of the body; solid wastes (feces) leave the body through the anus.

Aorta (a-OR-tah):   Largest artery, which leads from the lower left chamber of the heart to arteries all over the body.

Aortic stenosis (a-OR-tik steh-NO-sis):   Narrowing of the aorta.

Apex (A-peks):   Pointed end of an organ (pl. apices [A-pih-sez]).

Aphakia (ah-FA-ke-ah):   Absence of the lens of the eye.

Aphasia (ah-FA-ze-ah):   Absence or impairment of communication through speech.

Apnea (AP-ne-ah):   Not (A-) able to breathe (-PNEA).

Appendectomy (ap-en-DEK-to-me):   Removal of the appendix.

Appendicitis (ap-en-dih-SI-tis):   Inflammation of the appendix.

Appendix (ah-PEN-dikz):   Small sac that hangs from the juncture of the small and large intestines in the right lower quadrant of the abdomen. Its function is unknown.

Areola (ah-RE-o-lah):   Dark, pigmented area around the nipple of the breast.

Arrhythmia (a-RITH-me-ah):   Abnormal heart rhythm.

Arteriography (ar-ter-e-OG-ra-fe):   Process of recording (x-ray) of arteries after injecting contrast material.

Arteriole (ar-TER-e-ol):   Small artery.

Arteriolitis (ar-ter-e-o-LI-tis):   Inflammation of small arteries (arterioles).

Arteriosclerosis (ar-ter-e-o-skle-RO-sis):   Hardening of arteries. The most common form is *atherosclerosis,* which is hardening of arteries caused by collection of fatty, cholesterol-like deposits (plaque) in arteries.

Artery (AR-ter-e):   Largest blood vessel. Arteries carry blood away from the heart.

Arthralgia (ar-THRAL-je-ah):   Pain in a joint.

Arthritis (ar-THRI-tis):   Inflammation of a joint.

Arthrocentesis (ar-thro-sen-TE-sis):   Surgical puncture to remove fluid from a joint.

Arthrogram (AR-thro-gram):   X-ray record of a joint.

Arthropathy (ar-THROP-ah-the):   Disease of joints.

Arthroplasty (AR-thro-plas-te):   Surgical repair of a joint, especially to restore mobility in osteoarthritis or rheumatoid arthritis.

Arthroscope (AR-thro-skop):   Instrument used to examine the inside of a joint.

Arthroscopy (ar-THROS-ko-pe):   Process of visual examination of a joint.

Arthrosis (ar-THRO-sis):   Abnormal condition of a joint.

Ascites (ah-SI-tez):   Abnormal collection of fluid in the abdomen.

Asphyxia (as-FIK-se-ah):   Deficiency of oxygen in the blood and increase in carbon dioxide in blood and tissues. Major symptom is a complete absence of breathing.

AST: An enzyme normally present in blood and tissues such as heart and liver. Also called SGOT.

Asthma (AZ-mah):   Difficult breathing caused by a spasm of the bronchial tubes or a swelling of their mucous membrane lining.

Atelectasis (ah-teh-LEK-tah-sis):   Collapsed lung (ATEL-, meaning incomplete; -ECTASIS, meaning widening or dilation).

Atherosclerosis (ah-theh-ro-skle-RO-sis):   See ARTERIOSCLEROSIS.

Atrium (A-tre-um):   Upper chamber of the heart (pl. atria).

Atrophy (AT-ro-fe):   Decrease in size of cells within an organ.

Auditory canal (AW-dih-to-re kah-NAL):   Passageway leading into the ear from the outside of the body.

Auditory nerve (AW-dih-to-re nurve):   Nerve that carries messages from the inner ear to the brain, making hearing possible.

Aura (AW-rah):   A strange sensation coming before more definite symptoms of illness. An aura often precedes a migraine headache, warning the patient that an attack is beginning.

Aural discharge (AW-rah DIS-charge):   Fluid or material from the ear.

Autopsy (AW-top-se):   Examination of a dead body to determine the cause of death. Also called a postmortem exam or necropsy. Literally, it means "to see" (-OPSY) with "one's own" (AUT-) eyes.

Axial (AKS-e-al):   Pertaining to an axis (a line through the center of a body or about which a structure revolves).

Axillary (AKS-ih-lar-e):   Pertaining to the armpit or underarm.

B

Bactericidal (bak-tih-re-SI-dal):   Pertaining to an agent that destroys bacteria.

Bacteriostatic (bak-tih-re-o-STAT-ik):   Pertaining to an agent that inhibits bacterial growth.

Bacterium (bak-TIH-re-um):   Type of one-celled organism whose genetic material (DNA) is not organized within a nucleus (pl. bacteria).

Balanitis (bah-lah-NI-tis):   Inflammation of the penis.

Barium (BAH-re-um):   Substance used as a radiopaque (x-rays cannot pass through it) contrast medium for x-ray examination of the digestive tract.

Barium enema (BAH-re-um EN-eh-mah):   X-ray image of the lower digestive tract after injection of a solution of barium into the rectum.

Barium swallow (BAH-re-um SWA-lo):   X-ray image of the upper digestive tract after the patient swallows a solution of barium.

Benign (be-NIN):   Not cancerous; a tumor that does not spread and is limited in growth.

Benign prostatic hyperplasia (be-NIN pro-STAH-tik hi-per-PLA-ze- ah):   Nonmalignant enlargement of the prostate gland. Also called benign prostatic hypertrophy (hi-PER-tro-fe).

Benzodiazepine (be-zo-di-AZ-eh-pin):   Drug used to relieve anxiety, relax muscles, and produce sedation.

Beta blocker (BAY-tah BLOK-er):   Drug that is used for the treatment of high blood pressure (hypertension), chest pain (angina), and abnormal rhythms of the heart (arrhythmias).

Bilateral (bi-LAT-er-al):   Pertaining to two (both) sides.

Bile (bil):   A yellow or orange fluid produced by the liver. It breaks up large fat globules and helps the digestion of fats.

Bile duct (bil dukt):   Tube that carries bile from the liver and gallbladder to the intestine.

Bilirubin (bil-ih-RU-bin):   A red blood cell pigment excreted with bile from the liver into the intestine.

Biology (bi-OL-o-je):   Study of life.

Biopsy (BI-op-se):   Process of viewing living tissue with a microscope.

Bladder (BLAD-der):   See URINARY BLADDER.

Bone (bon):   Hard, rigid type of connective tissue that makes up most of the skeleton. It is composed of calcium salts.

Bone marrow (bon MAH-ro):   Soft, sponge-like material in the inner part of bones. Blood cells are made in the bone marrow.

Bradycardia (bra-de-KAR-de-ah):   Slow heartbeat.

Brain (bran):   Organ in the head that controls the activities of the body.

Breast (brest):   One of two glandular organs in front of the chest. The breasts produce milk after childbirth.

Bronchial tube (BRONG-ke-al tube):   One of two tubes that carry air from the windpipe to the lungs. Also called a bronchus (pl. bronchi).

Bronchiole (BRONG-ke-OL):   Small bronchial tube.

Bronchiolitis (brong-ke-o-LI-tis):   Inflammation of bronchioles.

Bronchitis (brong-KI-tis):   Inflammation of bronchial tubes.

Bronchoscope (BRONG-ko-skop):   Instrument used to visually examine bronchial tubes.

Bronchoscopy (brong-KOS-ko-pe):   Visual examination of bronchial tubes by passing an endoscope through the trachea (windpipe) into the bronchi.

Bronchus (BRONG-kus):   See BRONCHIAL TUBE.

Bursa (BUR-sah):   Sac of fluid near a joint (pl. bursae [BUR-see]).

Bursitis (bur-SI-tis):   Inflammation of a bursa.

C

Calcaneus (kal-KA-ne-us):   Heel bone.

Calcification (cal-sih-fih-KA-shun):   Accumulation of calcium salts in tissues.

Calcium channel blocker (KAL-se-um CHA-nal BLOK-er):   Drug that dilates arteries by inhibiting the flow of calcium into muscle cells that line arteries. It is used to treat hypertension (high blood pressure) and angina (chest pain caused by insufficient oxygen to heart muscle).

Calculus (KAL-ku-lus):   Stone (pl. calculi [KAL-ku-li]).

Callus (KA-us):   Bony deposit formed between and around the broken ends of a fractured bone. Also, a painless thickening of skin cells in areas of external pressure or friction.

Capillary (KAP-il-lar-e):   Smallest blood vessel (pl. capillaries).

Carbon dioxide (KAHR-bon di-OK-side):   Odorless, colorless gas formed in tissues and eliminated by the lungs.

Carcinoma (kar-sih-NO-mah):   Cancerous tumor. Carcinomas form from epithelial cells, which line the internal organs and cover the outside of the body.

Cardiac (KAR-de-ak):   Pertaining to the heart.

Cardiologist (kar-de-OL-o-jist):   Physician specializing in the study of the heart and heart disease.

Cardiology (kar-de-OL-o-je):   Study of the heart.

Cardiomegaly (kar-de-o-MEG-ah-le):   Enlargement of the heart.

Cardiomyopathy (kar-de-o-mi-OP-ah-the):   Disease of heart muscle.

Cardiovascular surgeon (kar-de-o-VAS-ku-lar SUR-jin):   Specialist in operating on the heart and blood vessels.

Cardioversion (KAR-de-o-ver-zhun):   Brief discharges of electricity passing across the chest to stop a cardiac ARRHYTHMIA. Also called defibrillation.

Carpals (KAR-palz):   Wrist bones.

Carpal tunnel syndrome (KAR-pal TUN-el SIN-drom):   Group of symptoms resulting from compression of the median nerve in the wrist. Symptoms include tingling, pain, and burning sensations in the hand and wrist.

Cartilage (KAR-tih-lij):   Flexible, fibrous connective tissue, found attached to the nose, ears, voice box, and windpipe and chiefly attached to bones at joints.

Cataract (KAT-ah-raht):   Clouding of the lens of the eye.

Cathartic (ka-THAR-tik):   Pertaining to a substance that causes the release of feces from the large intestine.

CAT scan (kat scan):   Computerized axial tomography. See CT SCAN.

Cell (sel):   Smallest unit or part of an organ.

Cellulitis (sel-u-LI-tis):   Inflammation of soft tissue under the skin; it is marked by swelling, redness, and pain and is caused by bacterial infection.

Cephalgia (seh-FAL-je-ah):   Headache. Shortened form of cephalalgia.

Cephalic (seh-FAL-ik):   Pertaining to the head.

Cephalosporin (sef-ah-lo-SPOR-in):   Antibiotic similar to penicillin and used to treat infections of the respiratory tract, ear, urinary tract, bones, and blood.

Cerebellar (ser-eh-BEL-ar):   Pertaining to the cerebellum.

Cerebellum (ser-eh-BEL-um):   Lower, back part of the brain that coordinates muscle movement and balance.

Cerebral (seh-RE-bral or SER-e-bral):   Pertaining to the CEREBRUM.

Cerebrovascular accident (seh-re-bro-VAS-ku-lar AK-sih-dent):   Disorder of blood vessels within the cerebrum. It results from inadequate blood supply to the brain. See also STROKE.

Cerebrum (seh-RE-brum):   Largest part of the brain. It controls thought processes, hearing, speech, vision, and body movements.

Cervical (SER-vi-kal):   Pertaining to the neck of the body or the neck (cervix) of the uterus.

Cervical region (SER-vi-kal RE-jin):   Seven backbones in the area of the neck.

Cervical vertebra (SER-vi-kal VER-teh-brah):   Backbone in the neck.

Cervix (SER-viks):   Lower, neck-like portion of the uterus opening into the vagina.

Cesarean section (seh-ZAR-re-an SEK-shun):   Incision of the uterus to remove the fetus at birth.

Chemotherapy (ke-mo-THER-ah-pe):   Treatment with drugs. Chemotherapy is most often used in the treatment for cancer.

Cholecystectomy (ko-le-sis-TEK-to-me):   Removal of the gallbladder.

Choledochoduodenostomy (ko-led-oh-ko-doo-o-deh-NOS-to-me):   New surgical attachment of the common bile duct to the duodenum; an anastomosis.

Choledochotomy (ko-led-o-KOT-o-me):   Incision of the common bile duct.

Cholelithiasis (ko-le-lih-THI-ah-sis):   Abnormal condition of gallstones.

Cholesterol (ko-LES-ter-ol):   Fatty substance made in the liver and found in the bloodstream. It is an important part of all cells and is necessary for creating hormones. It may accumulate in the lining of arteries, such as in the heart, causing heart disease, or in the gallbladder to form gallstones. Normal adult levels are 150 to 200 mg/dL.

Chondroma (kon-DRO-mah):   Benign tumor of cartilage.

Chondrosarcoma (kon-dro-sar-KO-mah):   Malignant tumor of CARTILAGE.

Chronic (KRON-ik):   Lasting a long time.

Chronic obstructive pulmonary disease (KRON-ik ob-STRUK-tiv PUL-mo-na-re dih-ZEZ):   Chronic limitation in airflow into and out of the body; includes chronic bronchitis, ASTHMA, and EMPHYSEMA.

Circulatory system (SER-ku-lah-tor-e SIS-tem):   Organs (heart and blood vessels) that carry blood throughout the body.

Cirrhosis (seh-RO-sis):   Liver disease with deterioration of the liver cells. Cirrhosis is often caused by alcoholism and poor nutrition.

Clavicle (KLAV-ih-kuhl):   Collar bone.

Clinical (KLIN-eh-kal):   Pertaining to the bedside or clinic; involving patient care.

Coccygeal (kok-sih-JE-al):   Pertaining to the tailbone (coccyx).

Coccygeal region (kok-sih-JE-al RE-jin):   Four fused (joined together) bones at the base of the spinal column (backbone).

Coccyx (KOK-siks):   Tailbone.

Colectomy (ko-LEK-to-me):   Removal of the colon (large intestine).

Colitis (ko-LI-tis):   Inflammation of the colon (large intestine).

Colocolostomy (ko-lo-ko-LOS-to-me):   New surgical connection between two previously unconnected portions of the colon. This is an anastomosis.

Colon (KO-lon):   Large intestine (bowel).

Colonic polyposis (ko-LON-ik pol-ih-PO-sis):   Growths or masses protruding from the mucous membrane lining the colon.

Colonoscopy (ko-lon-OS-ko-pe):   Visual examination of the colon.

Colorectal surgeon (ko-lo-REK-tal SUR-jin):   Physician specializing in operating on the colon and rectum.

Colostomy (ko-LOS-to-me):   Opening of the colon to the outside of the body.

Colposcopy (kol-POS-ko-pe):   Visual examination of the vagina and cervix.

Concussion (kon-KUS-un):   Loss of consciousness resulting from a blow to the head.

Congenital anomaly (con-JEN-ih-tal ah-NOM-ah-le):   See ANOMALY.

Congestive heart failure (kon-JES-tiv hart FAIL-ur):   Condition in which the heart is unable to pump its required amount of blood, resulting in inadequate oxygen to body cells.

Conization (ko-nih-ZA-shun):   Removal of a wedge-shaped piece (cone) of tissue from the cervix in the diagnosis and treatment of early cancer of the cervix.

Conjunctiva (kon-junk-TI-vah):   Thin protective membrane over the front of the eye and attached to the eyelids.

Conjunctivitis (kon-junk-ti-VI-tis):   Inflammation of the CONJUNCTIVA.

Connective tissue (kon-NEK-tiv TIS-u):   Fibrous tissue that supports and connects internal organs, bones, and walls of blood vessels.

Corium (KOR-e-um):   Middle layer of the skin below the epidermis; DERMIS.

Cornea (KOR-ne-ah):   Transparent layer over the front of the eye. It bends light to focus it on sensitive cells (retina) at the back of the eye.

Coronal plane (kor-O-nal playn):   See FRONTAL PLANE.

Coronary (KOR-on-ary):   Pertaining to the heart.

Coronary arteries (KOR-on-ary AR-ter-ez):   Blood vessels that carry oxygen-rich blood from the aorta to the heart muscle.

Cortex (KOR-teks):   Outer part of an organ (pl. cortices [KOR-teh-sez]).

Cortisol (KOR-tih-sol):   Anti-inflammatory hormone secreted by the adrenal cortex.

Costochondritis (kos-to-kon-DRI-tis):   Inflammation of a rib and its cartilage.

Costochondral (kos-to-KON-dral):   Pertaining to a rib and its cartilage.

Cranial cavity (KRA-ne-al KAV-ih-te):   Space surrounded by the skull and containing the brain and other organs.

Craniotomy (kra-ne-OT-o-me):   Incision of the skull.

Cranium (KRA-ne-um):   Skull.

Creatinine (kre-AT-tih-nin):   Nitrogen-containing waste that is removed from the blood by the kidney and excreted in urine.

Crohn disease (kron dih-ZEZ):   Inflammation of the gastrointestinal tract (often the ileum) marked by bouts of diarrhea, abdominal cramping, and fever. Along with ulcerative colitis, Crohn disease is a type of INFLAMMATORY BOWEL DISEASE.

Cross-section (kros SEK-shun):   Divides an organ or the body into upper and lower portions; TRANSVERSE PLANE.

Cryotherapy (kri-o-THER-ah-pe):   Treatment using cold (CRY/O) temperatures.

Cryptorchism (kript-OR-kism):   Undescended (CRYPT- means hidden) testicle. The testicle is not in the scrotal sac at birth.

CT scan: Computed tomography; series of x-ray images showing organs in cross-section (transverse view). Also called a CAT SCAN.

Cushing syndrome (KOOSH-ing SIN-drom):   Symptoms produced by an excess of cortisol from the adrenal cortex. Cushing syndrome is marked by moon face, fatty swellings, and weakness.

Cyanosis (si-ah-NO-sis):   Bluish discoloration of the skin due to deficient OXYGEN in the bloodstream.

Cystitis (sis-TI-tis):   Inflammation of the urinary bladder.

Cystoscope (SIS-to-skop):   Instrument (endoscope) used to view the urinary bladder.

Cystoscopy (sis-TOS-ko-pe):   Visual examination of the urinary bladder.

Cytology (si-TOL-o-je):   Study of cells.

𝒟

Debridement (de-BREED-ment):   Removal of diseased tissue from the skin.

Defibrillation (de-fib-rih-LA-shun):   Brief discharges of electricity applied to the chest to stop an abnormal heart rhythm.

Dementia (deh-MEN-shah):   Loss of memory and mental abilities.

Dermal (DER-mal):   Pertaining to the skin.

Dermatitis (der-mah-TI-tis):   Inflammation of the skin.

Dermatologist (der-mah-TOL-o-jist):   Physician specializing in the skin and its diseases.

Dermatology (der-mah-TOL-o-je):   Study of the skin and its diseases.

Dermatosis (der-mah-TO-sis):   Any abnormal condition of the skin.

Dermis (DER-mis):   Fibrous middle layer of the skin below the epidermis. The dermis contains nerves and blood vessels, hair roots, oil and sweat glands; the CORIUM.

Diabetes mellitus (di-ah-BE-tez MEL-li-tus):   Disorder marked by deficient insulin in the blood, which causes sugar to remain in the blood rather than entering cells. Diabetes is named from a Greek word meaning "siphon" (through which water passes easily). One symptom is frequent urination (polyuria). Type 1 diabetes is marked by lack of insulin, and patients need injections of insulin. In Type 2 diabetes, insulin is not adequately or appropriately secreted. Type 2 diabetes has a tendency to develop later in life, and patients are treated with diet, exercise, and oral antidiabetic drugs.

Diagnosis (di-ag-NO-sis):   Complete knowledge of patient's condition (pl. diagnoses).

Dialysis (di-AL-ih-sis):   Complete separation (-LYSIS) of wastes (urea) from the blood when the kidneys fail. See also HEMODIALYSIS and PERITONEAL DIALYSIS.

Diaphragm (DI-ah-fram):   Muscle that separates the chest from the abdomen.

Diarrhea (di-ah-RE-ah):   Discharge of watery wastes from the COLON.

Digestive system (di-JES-tiv SIS-tem):   Organs that bring food into the body and break it down to enter the bloodstream or eliminate it through the rectum and anus.

Dilation (di-LA-shun):   Widening; dilatation.

Dilation and curettage (di-LA-shun and kur-ih-TAJ):   Widening of the opening to the cervix and scraping (curettage) of the inner lining of the uterus; *D&C.*

Disk (disc):   Pad of cartilage that is between each backbone.

Diuretic (di-u-RET-ik):   Drug that causes kidneys to allow more fluid (as urine) to leave the body. Diuretics are used to treat HYPERTENSION. DI- (from DIA-) means complete, and UR- means urine.

Diverticula (di-ver-TIK-u-lah):   Small pouches or sacs created by herniation of mucous membrane linings, most commonly in the colon (sing. diverticulum).

Diverticulosis (di-ver-tik-u-LO-sis):   Abnormal condition of small pouches in the lining of the intestines.

Diverticulitis (di-ver-tik-u-LI-tis):   Inflammation of diverticula. Penetration of fecal material through thin-walled diverticula causes inflammation and infection in the colon.

Duodenal (do-o-DE-nal):   Pertaining to the duodenum.

Duodenum (do-o-DE-num):   First part of the small intestine.

Dysentery (DIS-en-teh-re):   Condition of painful intestines (often caused by bacterial infection).

Dysmenorrhea (dis-men-o-RE-ah):   Painful menstrual flow.

Dyspepsia (dis-PEP-se-ah):   Painful (DYS-) digestion (-PEPSIA).

Dysphagia (dis-FA-jah):   Difficult swallowing.

Dysphasia (dis-FA-zhah):   Difficult (impairment of) speech.

Dysplasia (dis-PLA-zhah):   Abnormality of the development or the formation of cells. Normal cells change in size, shape, and organization.

Dyspnea (disp-NE-ah):   Painful (DYS-) (labored, difficult) breathing (-PNEA).

Dysuria (dis-U-re-ah):   Painful or difficult urination.

E

Ear: Organ that receives sound waves and transmits them to nerves leading to the brain.

Eardrum (EAR-drum):   Membrane separating the outer and middle parts of the ear; the tympanic membrane.

Ectopic pregnancy (ek-TOP-ik PREG-nan-se):   Development of the zygote (early product of conception) in a place outside the uterus. The fallopian tubes are the most common ectopic site.

Edema (eh-DE-mah):   Swelling in tissues. Edema is often caused by retention (holding back) of fluid and salt by the kidneys.

Electrocardiogram (e-lek-tro-KAR-de-o-gram):   Record of the electricity in the heart.

Electroencephalogram (e-lek-tro-en-SEF-ah-lo-gram):   Record of the electricity in the brain.

Electroencephalography (e-lek-tro-en-sef-ah-LOG-ra-fe):   Process of recording the electricity in the brain.

Electrolyte (eh-LEK-tro-lite):   Substance (calcium, potassium, sodium) that conducts an electric current and is found in blood (serum) and body cells.

Embryo (EM-bre-o):   A new organism in an early stage of development (2 to 6 weeks). From 6 to 38 weeks, the developing infant is a FETUS.

Emergency medicine (e-MER-jen-se MED-ih-sin):   Care of patients requiring immediate action.

Emphysema (em-fih-SE-mah):   Lung disorder in which air becomes trapped in the air sacs and bronchioles, making breathing difficult. Emphysema is marked by the accumulation of mucus and the loss of elasticity in lung tissue.

Encephalitis (en-sef-ah-LI-tis):   Inflammation of the brain.

Encephalopathy (en-sef-ah-LOP-ah-the):   Disease of the brain.

Endocarditis (EN-do-kar-DI-tis):   Inflammation of the inner lining of the heart (endocardium).

Endocrine glands (EN-do-krin glanz):   Organs that produce (secrete) hormones.

Endocrine system (EN-do-krin SIS-tem):   Endocrine glands. Examples are the pituitary, thyroid, and adrenal glands and the pancreas.

Endocrinologist (en-do-krih-NOL-o-jist):   Specialist in the study of endocrine glands and their disorders.

Endocrinology (en-do-krih-NOL-o-je):   Study of ENDOCRINE GLANDS.

Endometriosis (en-do-me-tre-O-sis):   An abnormal condition in which tissue from the inner lining of the uterus is found outside the uterus, usually in the pelvic cavity.

Endometrium (en-do-ME-tre-um):   Inner lining of the uterus.

Endoscope (EN-do-skop):   Instrument used to view a hollow organ or body cavity; a tube fitted with a lens system that allows viewing in different directions.

Endoscopic retrograde cholangiopancreatography (en-do-SKOP-ik RET-tro-grade kol-an-je-o-pan-kre-ah-TOG-rah-fe):   X-ray images of bile ducts and pancreas after injection of contrast through a catheter from the mouth, esophagus, and stomach into bile and pancreatic ducts.

Endoscopy (en-DOS-ko-pe):   Process of viewing the inside of hollow organs or cavities with an endoscope.

Enteric (en-TER-ik):   Pertaining to the small intestine.

Enteritis (en-teh-RI-tis):   Inflammation of the small intestine.

Epidermis (ep-i-DER-mis):   Outer (EPI-) layer of the skin (-DERMIS).

Epidural hematoma (ep-ih-DUR-al he-mah-TO-mah):   Mass of blood above the dura mater (outermost layer of membranes surrounding the brain and spinal cord).

Epiglottis (ep-ih-GLOT-tis):   Flap of cartilage that covers the mouth of the trachea when swallowing occurs so that food cannot enter the airway.

Epiglottitis (ep-ih-glo-TI-tis):   Inflammation of the EPIGLOTTIS.

Epilepsy (EP-ih-lep-se):   Condition in which abnormal electrical activity in the brain results in sudden, fleeting disturbances in nerve cell functioning. An attack of epilepsy is called a SEIZURE.

Epinephrine (eh-pih-NEF-rin):   Hormone secreted by the adrenal gland in response to stress and physical injury. It is a drug used to treat hypersensitivity reactions (severe allergy), asthma, bronchial spasm, and nasal congestion. Also called ADRENALINE.

Epithelial (ep-ih-THE-le-al):   Pertaining to skin cells. This term originally described cells upon (EPI-) the breast nipple (THELI-). Now, it indicates cells lining the inner part of internal organs and covering the outside of the body.

Epithelium (ep-ih-THE-le-um):   Covering of the internal and external tissues of the body (skin, vessels, body cavities, glands, and organs).

Erythrocyte (eh-RITH-ro-site):   Red blood cell.

Erythrocytosis (eh-rith-ro-si-TO-sis):   Abnormal condition (slight increase in numbers) of red blood cells.

Erythromycin (eh-rith-ro-MI-sin):   An antibiotic that is produced from a red (ERYTHR/O-) mold (-MYCIN).

Esophageal (eh-sof-ah-JE-al):   Pertaining to the esophagus.

Esophagitis (eh-sof-ah-JI-tis):   Inflammation of the esophagus.

Esophagoscopy (eh-sof-ah-GOS-ko-pe):   Visual examination of the esophagus.

Esophagus (eh-SOF-ah-gus):   Tube leading from the throat to the stomach.

Estrogen (ES-tro-jen):   Hormone that promotes the development of female secondary sex characteristics. Examples are estradiol, estriol, and conjugated estrogen.

Eustachian tube (u-STA-she-an tube):   Channel connecting the middle part of the ear with the throat.

Excision (ek-SIZH-un):   Act of cutting out, removing, or resecting.

Exocrine glands (EK-so-krin glanz):   Glands that produce (secrete) chemicals that leave the body through tubes (ducts). Examples are tear, sweat, and salivary glands.

Exophthalmic goiter (ek-sof-THAL-mik GOY-ter):   Enlargement of the thyroid gland accompanied by high levels of thyroid hormone in the blood and protrusion of the eyeballs (EXOPHTHALMOS).

Exophthalmos (ek-sof-THAL-mos):   Abnormal protrusion of eyeballs usually caused by HYPERTHYROIDISM.

Extracranial (eks-tra-KRA-ne-al):   Pertaining to outside the skull.

Extrahepatic (eks-tra-heh-PAT-ik):   Pertaining to outside the liver.

Extrapulmonary (eks-trah-PUL-mo-nah-re):   Outside the lungs.

Eye (i):   Organ that receives light waves and transmits them to the brain.

𝓕

Fallopian tubes (fah-LO-pe-an tubz):   Two tubes that lead from the ovaries to the uterus. They transport egg cells to the uterus; also called uterine tubes.

Family medicine (FAM-i-le MED-ih-sin):   Primary care of all members of the family on a continuing basis.

Family practitioner (FAM-ih-le prak-TIH-shan-er):   Doctor responsible for primary care and treatment of patients on a continuing basis.

Fellowship training (FEL-o-ship TRA-ning):   Postgraduate training for doctors in specialized fields. The training may include CLINICAL and RESEARCH (laboratory) work.

Female reproductive system (FE-mal re-pro-DUK-tiv SIS-tem):   Organs (OVARIES) that produce and transport (FALLOPIAN TUBES) egg cells and secrete female hormones (ESTROGEN and PROGESTERONE). The system includes the uterus, where the embryo and fetus grow.

Femur (FE-mer):   Thigh bone.

Fetus (FE-tus):   Unborn offspring in the uterus after 8 weeks of pregnancy until birth.

Fibrillation (fih-brih-LA-shun):   Rapid, irregular, involuntary muscular contraction. Atrial and ventricular fibrillation are cardiac (heart) ARRHYTHMIAS.

Fibroid (FI-broyd):   Benign growth of muscle tissue in the uterus.

Fibrosarcoma (fi-bro-sar-KO-mah):   Malignant tumor of fibrous tissue.

Fibula (FIB-u-lah):   Smaller lower leg bone.

Fixation (fik-SA-shun):   Act of holding, sewing, or fastening a part in a fixed position.

Flutter (FLUT-er):   Rapid but regular, abnormal heart muscle contraction. Atrial and ventricular flutter are heart ARRHYTHMIAS.

Follicle-stimulating hormone (FOL-eh-kle STIM-u-la-ting HOR-mon):   A hormone secreted by the pituitary gland to stimulate the egg cells in the ovaries.

Fracture (FRAK-tur):   Breaking of a bone.

Frontal (FRUN-tal):   Pertaining to the front; anterior.

Frontal plane (FRUN-tal plan):   Imaginary line that divides an organ or the body into a front and back portion; the coronal plane.

G

Gallbladder (GAWL-bla-der):   Sac below the liver that stores bile and delivers it to the small intestine.

Ganglion (GANG-le-on):   Benign cyst near a joint (wrist); also, a group of nerve cells (pl. ganglia [GANG-le-ah]).

Gastralgia (gas-TRAL-jah):   Stomach pain.

Gastrectomy (gas-TREK-to-me):   Excision (removal) of the stomach.

Gastric (GAS-trik):   Pertaining to the stomach.

Gastritis (gas-TRI-tis):   Inflammation of the stomach.

Gastroenteritis (gas-tro-en-teh-RI-tis):   Inflammation of the stomach and intestines.

Gastroenterologist (gas-tro-en-ter-OL-o-jist):   Specialist in the treatment of stomach and intestinal disorders.

Gastroenterology (gas-tro-en-ter-OL-o-je):   Study of the stomach and intestines.

Gastroesophageal reflux disease (gas-tro-eh-sof-ah-JE-al RE-flux dih-ZEZ):   Backflow of contents of the stomach into the esophagus. Abbreviation is GERD.

Gastrojejunostomy (gas-tro-jeh-ju-NOS-to-me):   New surgical opening between the stomach and the jejunum (second part of the small intestine). This procedure is an anastomosis.

Gastroscope (GAS-tro-skop):   Instrument used to view the stomach. It is passed down the throat and esophagus into the stomach.

Gastroscopy (gas-TROS-ko-pe):   Visual examination of the stomach.

Gastrotomy (gas-TROT-o-me):   Incision of the stomach.

GERD: See GASTROESOPHAGEAL REFLUX DISEASE.

Geriatric (jer-e-AH-trik):   Pertaining to treatment of older people.

Geriatrician (jer-e-ah-TRISH-an):   Specialist in the treatment of diseases of old age.

Geriatrics (jer-e-AH-triks):   Treatment of disorders of old age.

Gestation (jes-TA-shun):   Pregnancy.

Gland: Group of cells that secretes chemicals to the outside of the body (EXOCRINE GLANDS) or hormones directly into the bloodstream (ENDOCRINE GLANDS).

Glaucoma (glaw-KO-mah):   Increase of fluid pressure within the eye. Fluid is formed more rapidly than it is removed. The increased pressure damages sensitive cells in the back of the eye, and vision is disturbed.

Glial cells (GLE-al sels):   Supporting cells of nervous tissue in the brain. Examples are astrocytes, microglial and oligodendroglial cells. These cells are the source of primary brain tumors.

Glioblastoma (gli-o-blas-TO-mah):   Malignant brain tumor composed of immature (-BLAST) glial (supportive nervous tissue) cells.

Glucocorticoid (gloo-ko-KOR-tih-koid):   Hormone secreted by the adrenal gland (cortex) to raise blood sugar levels. Examples are cortisone and cortisol.

Glycosuria (gli-ko-SU-re-ah):   Abnormal condition of sugar in the urine.

Goiter (GOY-ter):   Enlargement of the thyroid gland.

Gout (gout):   See GOUTY ARTHRITIS.

Gouty arthritis (gowti arth-RI-tis):   Deposits of uric acid crystals in joints and other tissues that cause swelling and inflammation of joints. Also called gout.

Graves disease (gravs dih-ZEZ):   See HYPERTHYROIDISM.

Growth hormone (groth HOR-mon):   Hormone secreted by the pituitary gland to stimulate the growth of bones and the body in general. Also called somatotropin.

Gynecologist (gi-neh-KOL-o-jist):   Specialist in the medical and surgical treatment of female disorders.

Gynecology (gi-neh-KOL-o-je):   Study of female disorders.

H

Hair follicle (hahr FOL-ih-kl):   Pouch-like depression in the skin in which a hair develops.

Hair root (hahr root):   Part of the hair from which growth occurs.

HDL: See HIGH-DENSITY LIPOPROTEIN.

Heart (hart):   Hollow, muscular organ in the chest that pumps blood throughout the body.

Heart attack (hart a-TAK):   See MYOCARDIAL INFARCTION.

Hemangioma (he-man-je-O-mah):   Tumor (benign) of blood vessels.

Hematemesis (he-mah-TEM-eh-sis):   Vomiting (-EMESIS) of blood (HEMAT/O-).

Hematologist (he-mah-TOL-o-jist):   Specialist in blood and blood disorders.

Hematology (he-mah-TOL-o-je):   Study of the blood.

Hematoma (he-mah-TO-mah):   Mass or collection of blood under the skin. Commonly called a bruise or "black-and-blue" mark.

Hematuria (he-mah-TUR-e-ah):   Abnormal condition of blood in the urine.

Hemigastrectomy (heh-me-gas-TREK-to-me):   Removal of half of the stomach.

Hemiglossectomy (hem-e-glos-EK-to-me):   Removal of half of the tongue.

Hemiplegia (hem-ih-PLE-jah):   Paralysis of one side of the body.

Hemodialysis (he-mo-di-AL-ih-sis):   Use of a kidney machine to filter blood to remove waste materials such as urea. Blood leaves the body, enters the machine, and is carried back to the body through a catheter (tube).

Hemoglobin (HE-mo-glo-bin):   Oxygen-carrying protein found in red blood cells.

Hemoptysis (he-MOP-tih-sis):   Spitting up (-PTYSIS) of blood (HEM/O-).

Hemorrhage (HEM-or-ij):   Bursting forth of blood.

Hemothorax (he-mo-THOR-aks):   Collection of blood in the chest (pleural cavity).

Hepatic (heh-PAT-ik):   Pertaining to the liver.

Hepatitis (hep-ah-TI-tis):   Inflammation of the liver. Viral hepatitis is an acute infectious disease caused by at least three different viruses: hepatitis A, B, and C viruses.

Hepatoma (hep-ah-TO-mah):   Tumor (malignant) of the liver; hepatocellular carcinoma.

Hepatomegaly (hep-ah-to-MEG-ah-le):   Enlargement of the liver.

Hernia (HER-ne-ah):   Bulge or protrusion of an organ or part of an organ through the wall of the cavity that usually contains it. In an INGUINAL hernia, part of the wall of the abdomen weakens and the intestine bulges out or into the SCROTAL sac (in males).

Hiatal hernia (hi-A-tal HER-ne-ah):   Upward protrusion of the wall of the stomach into the lower part of the esophagus.

High-density lipoprotein (hi-DEN-sih-te li-po-PRO-teen):   Combination of fat and protein in the blood. It carries cholesterol to the liver, which is beneficial.

HIV: See HUMAN IMMUNODEFICIENCY VIRUS.

Hodgkin disease (HOJ-kin di-ZEZ):   Malignant tumor of lymph nodes.

Hormone (HOR-mon):   Chemical made by a gland and sent directly into the bloodstream, not to the outside of the body. ENDOCRINE GLANDS produce hormones.

Human immunodeficiency virus (U-man im-u-no-deh-FISH-en-se VI-rus):   Virus that infects white blood cells (T cell lymphocytes), causing damage to the patient's immune system. HIV is the cause of AIDS.

Humerus (HU-mer-us):   Upper arm bone.

Hydrocele (HI-dro-sel):   Swelling of the SCROTUM caused by a collection of fluid within the outermost covering of the TESTIS.

Hyperbilirubinemia (hi-per-bil-e-roo-bin-E-me-ah):   High levels of bilirubin (pigment released from hemoglobin breakdown and processed in the liver) in the bloodstream. See JAUNDICE.

Hyperglycemia (hi-per-gli-SE-me-ah):   Higher than normal levels of sugar in the blood.

Hyperparathyroidism (hi-per-par-ah-THI-royd-ism):   Higher than normal level of parathyroid hormone in the blood.

Hyperplastic (hi-per-PLAS-tik):   Pertaining to excessive growth of normal cells in an organ.

Hypersecretion (hi-per-se-KRE-shun):   An abnormally high amount of production of a substance.

Hypertension (hi-per-TEN-shun):   High blood pressure. *Essential hypertension* has no known cause, but contributing factors are age, obesity, smoking, and heredity. *Secondary hypertension* is a symptom of other disorders such as kidney disease.

Hyperthyroidism (hi-per-THI-royd-izm):   Excessive activity of the thyroid gland.

Hypertrophy (hi-PER-tro-fe):   Enlargement or overgrowth of an organ or part of the body as a result of an increase in size of individual cells.

Hypochondriac (hi-po-KON-dre-ak):   Pertaining to lateral regions of the upper abdomen beneath the lower ribs. Also, the term describes a person who has chronic concern about the health of his/her body.

Hypodermic (hi-po-DER-mik):   Pertaining to under or below the skin.

Hypoglycemia (hi-po-gli-SE-me-ah):   Blood condition of decreased sugar (lower than normal levels).

Hypophyseal (hi-po-FIZ-e-al):   Pertaining to the pituitary gland.

Hypopituitarism (hi-po-pi-TU-ih-tah-rizm):   Decrease or stoppage of hormonal secretion by the pituitary gland.

Hypoplastic (hi-po-PLAS-tik):   Pertaining to underdevelopment of a tissue or organ in the body.

Hyposecretion (hi-po-se-KRE-shun):   Less than normal amount of production of a substance.

Hypotensive (hi-po-TEN-siv):   Pertaining to low blood pressure or to a person with abnormally low blood pressure.

Hypothyroidism (hi-po-THI-royd-izm):   Lower than normal activity of the thyroid gland.

Hysterectomy (his-teh-REK-to-me):   Excision of the uterus, either through the abdominal wall (abdominal hysterectomy) or through the vagina (vaginal hysterectomy).

Hysteroscopy (his-ter-OS-ko-pe):   Visual examination of the uterus with an endoscope inserted through the vagina.

I

Iatrogenic (i-ah-tro-JEN-ik):   Pertaining to a patient's abnormal condition that results unexpectedly from a specific treatment.

Ileostomy (il-e-OS-to-me):   New opening of the ileum (third part of the small intestine) to the outside of the body.

Ileum (IL-e-um):   Third part of the small intestine.

Ilium (IL-e-um):   Side, high portion of the hip bone (pelvis).

Incision (in-SIZH-un):   Cutting into the body or into an organ.

Infarction (in-FARK-shun):   Area of dead tissue (necrosis) caused by decreased blood flow to that part of the body.

Infectious disease specialist (in-FEK-shus dih-ZEZ SPESH-ah-list):   Physician who treats disorders caused and spread by microorganisms such as bacteria.

Infiltrate (IN-fil-trat):   Material that accumulates in an organ. The term infiltrate often describes solid material and fluid collection in the lungs.

Inflammatory bowel disease (in-FLAM-ah-to-re BOW-el dih-ZEZ):   Disorder of the small and large intestines marked by bouts of diarrhea, abdominal cramping, and fever. Inflammatory bowel diseases include CROHN DISEASE and ULCERATIVE COLITIS.

Inguinal (ING-gwi-nal):   Pertaining to the groin or the area where the legs meet the body.

Insulin (IN-su-lin):   Hormone produced by the pancreas and released into the bloodstream. Insulin allows sugar to leave the blood and enter body cells.

Internal medicine (in-TER-nal MED-ih-sin):   Branch of medicine specializing in the diagnosis of disorders and treatment with drugs.

Intervertebral (in-ter-VER-teh-bral):   Pertaining to lying between two backbones. A disk (disc) is an intervertebral structure.

Intra-abdominal (in-trah-ab-DOM-ih-nal):   Pertaining to within the abdomen.

Intracranial (in-tra-KRA-ne-al):   Pertaining to within the skull.

Intrauterine (in-trah-U-ter-in):   Pertaining to within the uterus.

Intravenous (in-trah-VE-nus):   Pertaining to within a vein.

Intravenous pyelogram (in-trah-VEN-nus PI-eh-lo-gram):   X-ray record of the kidney (PYEL/O- means renal pelvis) after contrast is injected into a vein.

Iris (I-ris):   Colored (pigmented) portion of the eye.

Ischemia (is-KE-me-ah):   Deficiency of blood flow to a part of the body, caused by narrowing or obstruction of blood vessels.

J

Jaundice (JAWN-dis):   Orange-yellow coloration of the skin and other tissues. A symptom caused by accumulation of BILIRUBIN (pigment) in the blood.

Jejunum (jeh-JE-num):   Second part of the small intestine.

Joint (joynt):   Space where two or more bones come together (articulate).

K

Kidney (KID-ne):   One of two organs behind the abdomen that produce urine by filtering wastes from the blood.

L

Laminectomy (lah-men-EK-to-me):   Removal of a piece of backbone (lamina) to relieve pressure on nerves from a herniating disk (disc).

Laparoscope (LAP-ah-ro-skop):   Instrument to visually examine the abdomen. An endoscope is inserted through a small incision in the abdominal wall.

Laparoscopic appendectomy (lap-ah-ro-SKOP-ik ah-pen-DEK-to-me):   Removal of the appendix through a small incision in the abdomen and with the use of a laparoscope.

Laparoscopic cholecystectomy (lap-ah-ro-SKOP-ik ko-le-sis-TEK-to-me):   Removal of the gallbladder through a small incision in the abdomen and with the use of a laparoscopic instrument.

Laparoscopy (lap-ah-ROS-ko-pe):   Visual examination of the abdomen. A small incision is made near the navel, and an instrument (endoscope) is inserted to view abdominal organs.

Laparotomy (lap-ah-ROT-o-me):   Incision of the abdomen. A surgeon makes a large incision across the abdomen to examine and operate on its organs.

Large intestine (larj in-TES-tin):   Part of the intestine that receives undigested material from the small intestine and transports it out of the body; the COLON.

Laryngeal (lah-rin-JE-al):   Pertaining to the larynx (voice box).

Laryngectomy (lah-rin-JEK-to-me):   Removal of the larynx (voice box).

Laryngitis (lah-rin-JI-tis):   Inflammation of the larynx.

Laryngoscopy (lar-in-GOS-ko-pe):   Visual examination of the interior of the voice box (larynx) with an endoscope.

Laryngotracheitis (lah-ring-o-tra-ke-I-tis):   Inflammation of the larynx and the trachea (windpipe).

Larynx (LAR-inks):   Voice box; located at the top of the trachea and containing vocal cords.

Lateral (LAT-er-al):   Pertaining to the side.

LDL: See LOW-DENSITY LIPOPROTEIN.

Leiomyoma (li-o-mi-O-mah):   Benign tumor derived from smooth (involuntary) muscle and most often of the uterus (leiomyoma uteri). LEIOMY/O- means smooth, visceral, or involuntary muscle.

Leiomyosarcoma (li-o-mi-o-sar-KO-mah):   Malignant tumor of smooth (involuntary) muscle.

Lens (lenz):   Structure behind the pupil of the eye. The lens bends light rays so that they are properly focused on the RETINA at the back of the eye.

Lesion (LE-zhun):   Damage to a part of the body, caused by disease or trauma.

Leukemia (lu-KE-me-ah):   Increase in malignant (cancerous) white blood cells in blood and bone marrow.

Leukocyte (LOO-ko-sit):   White blood cell.

Leukocytosis (lu-ko-si-TO-sis):   Slight increase in the numbers of normal white blood cells as a response to infection.

Ligament (LIG-ah-ment):   Connective tissue that joins bones to other bones.

Ligamentous (lig-ah-MEN-tus):   Pertaining to a LIGAMENT.

Liposarcoma (li-po-sar-KO-mah):   Malignant tumor of fatty tissue.

Lithotripsy (LITH-o-trip-se):   Process of crushing a stone in the urinary tract using ultrasonic vibrations. Also called extracorporeal shock-wave lithotripsy (ESWL).

Liver (LIV-er):   Organ in the right upper quadrant of the abdomen. The liver produces BILE, stores sugar, and produces blood-clotting proteins.

Lobe (lob):   Part of an organ, especially of the brain, lungs, or glands.

Low-density lipoprotein (lo-DEN-sih-te li-po-PRO-teen):   Combination of lipid (fat) and protein. It has a high CHOLESTEROL content and is associated with forming plaques in arteries.

Lower gastrointestinal (GI) series (LOW-er gas-tro-in-TES-tin-al SER-ez):   Barium is injected into the anus and rectum and x-rays are taken of the colon (large intestine).

Lumbar (LUM-bar):   Pertaining to the loins; part of the back and sides between the chest and the hip.

Lumbar region (LUM-bar RE-jin):   Pertaining to the backbones that lie between the thoracic (chest) and sacral (lower back) vertebrae.

Lumbar vertebra (LUM-bar VER-teh-brah):   A backbone in the region between the chest and lower back.

Lung (lung):   One of two paired organs in the chest through which oxygen enters and carbon dioxide leaves the body.

Lung capillaries (lung KAP-ih-lar-ez):   Tiny blood vessels surrounding lung tissue and through which gases pass into and out of the bloodstream.

Lupus erythematosus: See SYSTEMIC LUPUS ERYTHEMATOSUS.

Lymph (limf):   Clear fluid that is found in lymph vessels and produced from fluid surrounding cells. Lymph contains white blood cells (lymphocytes) that fight disease.

Lymphadenectomy (limf-ah-deh-NEK-to-me):   Removal of LYMPH NODES.

Lymphadenopathy (lim-fad-eh-NOP-ah-the):   Disease of lymph nodes (glands).

Lymphangiectasis (limf-an-je-EK-tah-sis):   Dilation (-ECTASIS) of small lymph vessels; often resulting from obstruction in large lymph vessels.

Lymphatic system (lim-FAT-ik SIS-tem):   Group of organs (lymph vessels, lymph nodes, spleen, thymus) composed of lymphatic tissue that produce lymphocytes to defend the body against foreign organisms.

Lymphatic vessels (lim-FAT-ik VES-elz):   Tubes that carry lymph from tissues to the bloodstream (into a vein in the neck region); lymph vessels.

Lymphedema (limf-ah-DE-mah):   Accumulation of fluid in tissue spaces, causing swelling. Lymphedema is caused by the obstruction of lymph nodes or vessels.

Lymph node (limf nod):   Stationary collection of lymph cells, found all over the body. Lymph nodes are sometimes called lymph "glands."

Lymphocyte (LIMF-o-site):   White blood cell that is found within lymph and lymph nodes. T cells and B cells are types of lymphocytes.

Lymphoid (LIM-foid):   Resembling or pertaining to lymph tissue.

Lymphoma (lim-FO-mah):   Malignant tumor of lymphatic tissue. Previously called lymphosarcoma. There are several types, including Hodgkin disease and non-Hodgkin lymphoma.

M

Magnetic resonance imaging (mag-NET-ik REZ-o-nans IM-aj-ing):   Image of the body with magnetic and radio waves. Organs are seen in three planes: coronal (front to back), sagittal (side to side), and transverse (cross-section). Called *MRI*.

Male reproductive system (mal re-pro-DUK-tiv SIS-tem):   Organs that produce sperm cells and male hormones.

Malignant (mah-LIG-nant):   Tending to become progressively worse. The term malignant describes cancerous tumors that invade and spread to distant organs.

Mammary (MAM-er-e):   Pertaining to the breast.

Mammogram (MAM-o-gram):   X-ray record of the breast.

Mammography (mam-MOG-ra-fe):   Process of making an x-ray recording of the breast.

Mammoplasty (MAM-o-plas-te):   Surgical repair (reconstruction) of the breast.

Mastectomy (mas-TEK-to-me):   Removal (excision) of the breast.

Mastitis (mas-TI-tis):   Inflammation of the breast.

Mediastinal (me-de-ah-STI-nal):   Pertaining to the MEDIASTINUM.

Mediastinoscopy (me-de-ah-sti-NOS-ko-pe):   Visual examination of the mediastinum with an endoscope.

Mediastinum (me-de-ah-STI-num):   Space between the lungs in the chest. The mediastinum contains the heart, large blood vessels, trachea, esophagus, thymus gland, and lymph nodes.

Medulla oblongata (meh-DUL-ah ob-lon-GA-tah):   Lower part of the brain near the spinal cord. The medulla oblongata controls breathing and heartbeat.

Medullary (MEH-DU-lar-e):   Pertaining to the inner, or soft, part of an organ.

Melanoma (meh-lah-NO-mah):   Malignant tumor arising from pigmented cells (melanocytes) in the skin. A melanoma usually develops from a NEVUS (mole).

Meninges (meh-NIN-jes):   Membranes surrounding the brain and spinal cord.

Meningitis (men-in-JI-tis):   Inflammation of the meninges (membranes around the brain and spinal cord).

Menorrhagia (men-or-RA-jah):   Excessive bleeding from the uterus during the time of MENSTRUATION.

Menorrhea (men-o-RE-ah):   Normal discharge of blood and tissue from the uterine lining during MENSTRUATION.

Menses (MEN-sez):   Menstruation; menstrual period.

Menstruation (men-stru-A-shun):   Breakdown of the lining of the uterus that occurs every 4 weeks during the active reproductive period of a female.

Mesothelioma (mes-o-the-le-O-mah):   Malignant tumor of the lining tissue (mesothelium) of the pleura. A mesothelioma is associated with exposure to asbestos.

Metacarpals (met-ah-KAR-palz):   Bones of the hand between the wrist bones (carpals) and the finger bones (phalanges).

Metastasis (meh-TAS-tah-sis):   Spread of a cancerous tumor to a distant organ or location. Metastasis literally means change (META-) of place (-STASIS). *Metastatic* means pertaining to a metastasis.

Metatarsals (meh-tah-TAR-sels):   Foot bones.

Migraine (MI-gran):   Attack of headache, usually on one side of the head, caused by changes in blood vessel size and accompanied by nausea, vomiting, and sensitivity to light (photophobia). Migraine is a term from the French word *migraine,* meaning "severe head pain."

Minimally invasive surgery (MIN-ih-mal-le in-VA-siv SUR-jer-e):   Removal and repair of organs and tissues with small incisions for an endoscope and instruments. Examples are laparoscopic cholecystectomy (gallbladder removal), laparoscopic appendectomy (appendix removal), laparoscopic herniorrhaphy (repair of a hernia), and laparoscopic colectomy (removal of a portion of the colon).

Monocyte (MON-o-sit):   White blood cell with one large nucleus.

Mononucleosis (mon-o-nu-kle-O-sis):   An acute infectious disease with excess monocytes in the blood. Mononucleosis is caused by the Epstein-Barr virus and is transmitted by direct oral (mouth) contact.

Mouth (mowth):   The opening that forms the beginning of the digestive system.

MRI: See MAGNETIC RESONANCE IMAGING.

Multiple myeloma (MUL-tih-pul mi-eh-LO-mah):   Malignant tumor of the bone marrow.

Multiple sclerosis (MUL-tih-pul skeh-RO-sis):   Chronic neurological disease in which there are patches of demyelination (loss of myelin sheath covering on nerve cells) throughout the brain and spinal cord. Weakness, abnormal sensations, incoordination, and speech and visual disturbances are symptoms.

Muscle (MUS-el):   Connective tissue that contracts to make movement possible.

Muscular (MUS-ku-lar):   Pertaining to muscles.

Muscular dystrophy (MUS-ku-lar DIS-tro-fe):   Group of degenerative muscle diseases that cause crippling because muscles are gradually weakened and eventually ATROPHY (shrink).

Musculoskeletal system (mus-ku-lo-SKEL-e-tal SIS-tem):   Organs that support the body and allow it to move, including the muscles, bones, joints, and connective tissues.

Myalgia (mi-AL-jah):   Pain in a muscle or muscles.

Myelin sheath (MI-eh-lin sheth):   Fatty covering around part (axon) of nerve cells. The myelin sheath insulates and speeds the conduction of nerve impulses.

Myelodysplasia (mi-eh-lo-dis-PLA-ze-ah):   Abnormal development of bone marrow, a premalignant condition leading to leukemia.

Myelogram (MI-eh-lo-gram):   X-ray image of the spinal cord after contrast is injected within the membranes surrounding the spinal cord in the lumbar area of the back.

Myelography (mi-eh-LOG-rah-fe):   X-ray imaging of the spinal cord after injection of contrast material.

Myeloma (mi-eh-LO-mah):   Malignant tumor originating in the bone marrow (MYEL/O-). Also called MULTIPLE MYELOMA.

Myocardial (mi-o-KAR-de-al):   Pertaining to the muscle of the heart.

Myocardial infarction (mi-o-KAR-de-al in-FARK-shun):   Area of dead tissue in heart muscle; also known as a heart attack or an MI.

Myocardial ischemia (mi-o-KAR-de-al is-KE-me-ah):   Decrease in the blood supply to the heart muscle.

Myoma (mi-O-mah):   Tumor (benign) of muscle.

Myomectomy (mi-o-MEK-to-me):   Removal of a benign muscle tumor (fibroid).

Myosarcoma (mi-o-sar-KO-mah):   Tumor (malignant) of muscle. SARC- means flesh, indicating that the tumor is of connective or "fleshy" tissue origin.

Myositis (mi-o-SI-tis):   Inflammation of a muscle.

Myringotomy (mir-in-GOT-o-me):   Incision of the eardrum.

Nasal (NA-zel):   Pertaining to the nose.

Nausea (NAW-se-ah):   Unpleasant sensation in the upper abdomen, often leading to vomiting. The term comes from the Greek *nausia,* meaning "sea sickness."

Necrosis (neh-KRO-sis):   Death of cells.

Necrotic (neh-KRO-tik):   Pertaining to death of cells.

Neonatal (ne-o-NA-tal):   Pertaining to new birth; the first 4 weeks after birth.

Neoplasm (NE-o-plazm):   Any new growth of tissue; a tumor.

Neoplastic (ne-o-PLAS-tik):   Pertaining to a new growth, or NEOPLASM.

Nephrectomy (neh-FREK-to-me):   Removal (excision) of a kidney.

Nephritis (neh-FRI-tis):   Inflammation of kidneys.

Nephrolithiasis (neh-fro-lih-THI-ah-sis):   Condition of kidney stones.

Nephrologist (neh-FROL-o-jist):   Specialist in the diagnosis and treatment of kidney diseases.

Nephrology (neh-FROL-o-je):   Study of the kidney and its diseases.

Nephropathy (neh-FROP-ah-the):   Disease of the kidney.

Nephrosis (neh-FRO-sis):   Abnormal condition of the kidney. Nephrosis is often associated with a deterioration of the kidney tubules.

Nephrostomy (neh-FROS-to-me):   Opening from the kidney to the outside of the body.

Nervous system (NER-vus SIS-tem):   Organs (brain, spinal cord, and nerves) that transmit electrical messages throughout the body.

Neural (NU-ral):   Pertaining to nerves.

Neuralgia (nu-RAL-jah):   Nerve pain.

Neuritis (nu-RI-tis):   Inflammation of a nerve.

Neuroglial cells (nu-ro-GLE-al selz):   See GLIAL CELLS.

Neurologist (nu-ROL-o-jist):   Specialist in the diagnosis and treatment of nervous disorders.

Neurology (nu-ROL-o-je):   Study of the nervous system and nerve disorders.

Neuropathy (nu-ROP-ah-the):   Disease of nervous tissue.

Neurosurgeon (nu-ro-SUR-jin):   Physician who operates on the organs of the nervous system (brain, spinal cord, and nerves).

Neurotomy (nu-ROT-o-me):   Incision of a nerve.

Nevus (NE-vus):   Pigmented lesion on the skin; a mole.

Nocturia (nok-TU-re-ah):   Excessive urination at night.

Nose (noz):   Structure that is the organ of smell and permits air to enter and leave the body.

Nosocomial (nos-o-KO-me-al):   Pertaining to or originating in a hospital. A nosocomial infection is acquired during hospitalization.

O

Obstetric (ob-STEH-TRIK):   Pertaining to pregnancy, labor, and delivery of a baby.

Obstetrician (ob-steh-TRISH-un):   Specialist in the delivery of a baby and care of the mother during pregnancy and labor.

Obstetrics (ob-STET-riks):   Practice or branch of medicine concerned with the management of women during pregnancy, childbirth, and the period just after delivery of the infant.

Ocular (OK-u-lar):   Pertaining to the eye.

Oncogenic (ong-ko-JEN-ik):   Pertaining to producing (-GENIC) tumors.

Oncologist (ong-KOL-o-jist):   Physician specializing in the study and treatment of tumors.

Oncology (ong-KOL-o-je):   Study of tumors.

Oocyte (o-o-sit):   Egg cell (ovum).

Oophorectomy (o-of-o-REK-to-me or oo-fo-REK-to-me):   Removal of an ovary or ovaries.

Oophoritis (o-of-o-RI-tis or oo-pho-RI-tis):   Inflammation of an ovary.

Ophthalmologist (of-thal-MOL-o-jist):   Specialist in the study of the eye and the treatment of eye disorders.

Ophthalmology (of-thal-MOL-o-je):   Study of the eye; the diagnosis and treatment of eye disorders.

Ophthalmoscope (of-THAL-mo-scop):   Instrument used to visually examine the eye.

Optic nerve (OP-tik nerv):   Nerve in the back of the eye that transmits light waves to the brain.

Optician (op-TISH-an):   Nonmedical specialist trained to provide eyeglasses by filling prescriptions.

Optometrist (op-TOM-eh-trist):   Nonmedical specialist trained to examine and test eyes and prescribe corrective lenses.

Oral (OR-al):   Pertaining to the mouth.

Orchidectomy (or-kih-DEK-to-me):   Removal (excision) of a testicle or testicles.

Orchiectomy (or-ke-EK-to-me):   Removal (excision) of a testicle or testicles.

Orchiopexy (or-ke-o-PEK-se):   Surgical fixation of the testicle (testis) into its proper location within the scrotum. This surgery corrects CRYPTORCHISM.

Orchitis (or-KI-tis):   Inflammation of a testicle.

Organ (OR-gan):   Independent part of the body composed of different tissues working together to do a specific job.

Orthopedist (or-tho-PE-dist):   Specialist in the surgical correction of musculoskeletal disorders. This physician was originally concerned with straightening (ORTH/O-) bones in the legs of deformed children (PED/O-).

Osteitis (os-te-I-tis):   Inflammation of a bone.

Osteoarthritis (os-te-o-ar-THRI-tis):   Inflammation of bones and joints. Osteoarthritis is a disease of older people and is marked by stiffness, pain, and degeneration of joints.

Osteogenic sarcoma (os-te-o-JEN-ik sar-KO-mah):   Malignant (cancerous) tumor of bone (-GENIC means produced in).

Osteoma (os-te-O-mah):   Tumor (benign) of bone.

Osteomyelitis (os-te-o-mi-eh-LI-tis):   Inflammation of bone and bone marrow. Osteomyelitis is caused by a bacterial infection.

Osteopenia (os-te-o-PE-ne-ah):   Deficiency (-PENIA) of bone tissue.

Osteoporosis (os-te-o-po-RO-sis):   Decrease in bone mass with formation of pores or spaces in normally mineralized bone tissue.

Osteotomy (os-te-OT-o-me):   Incision of a bone.

Otalgia (o-TAL-jah):   Pain in an ear.

Otitis (o-TI-tis):   Inflammation of an ear.

Otolaryngologist (o-to-lah-rin-GOL-o-jist):   Specialist in the treatment of diseases of the ear, nose, and throat.

Ovarian (o-VAR-e-an):   Pertaining to an ovary or ovaries.

Ovarian cancer (o-VAR-e-an KAN-ser):   Malignant condition of the ovaries.

Ovarian cyst (o-VAR-e-an sist):   Sac containing fluid or semisolid material in or on the ovary.

Ovary (O-vah-re):   One of two organs in the female abdomen that produces egg cells and female hormones.

Ovum (O-vum):   Egg cell (pl. ova [o-VAH]).

Oxygen (OK-si-jen):   Colorless, odorless gas that is essential to sustaining life.

P

Pancreas (PAN-kre-us):   Gland that produces digestive juices (exocrine function) and the hormone INSULIN (endocrine function).

Pancreatectomy (pan-kre-ah-TEK-to-me):   Removal of the pancreas.

Pancreatitis (pan-kre-ah-TI-tis):   Inflammation of the pancreas.

Paralysis (pah-RAL-ih-sis):   Loss or impairment of movement in a part of the body.

Paraplegia (par-ah-PLE-jah):   Impairment or loss of movement in the lower part of the body, primarily the legs and in some cases bowel and bladder function.

Parathyroid glands (par-ah-THI-royd glanz):   Four endocrine glands behind the thyroid gland. These glands are concerned with maintaining the proper levels of calcium in the blood and bones.

Parathyroid hormone (par-ah-THI-roid HOR-mon):   Hormone secreted by the parathyroid glands to maintain a constant concentration of calcium in the blood and bones. Also called PTH.

Patella (pah-TEL-ah):   Knee cap.

Pathologist (pah-THOL-o-jist):   Specialist in the study of disease using microscopic examination of tissues and cells and autopsy examination.

Pathology (pah-THOL-o-je):   Study of disease.

Pediatric (pe-de-AT-rik):   Pertaining to treatment of a child.

Pediatrician (pe-de-ah-TRISH-un):   Specialist in the treatment of childhood diseases.

Pediatrics (pe-de-AT-riks):   Branch of medicine specializing in the treatment of children.

Pelvic (PEL-vik):   Pertaining to the bones of the hip area.

Pelvic cavity (PEL-vik KAV-ih-te):   Space contained within the hip bones (front and sides) and the lower part of the backbone (sacrum and coccyx).

Pelvic inflammatory disease (PEL-vik in-FLAM-ah-to-re dih-ZEZ):   Inflammation in the pelvic region; usually inflammation of the fallopian tubes.

Pelvis (PEL-vis):   Lower part of the trunk of the body including the hip bone, tailbone, and sacrum (lower backbones).

Penicillin (pen-ih-SIL-in):   Substance, derived from certain molds, that can destroy bacteria; an ANTIBIOTIC.

Penis (PE-nis):   External male organ containing the urethra, through which both urine and semen (sperm cells and fluid) leave the body.

Peptic ulcer (PEP-tik UL-ser):   Sore (lesion) of the mucous membrane lining the first part of the small intestine (duodenum) or lining the stomach.

Percutaneous (per-ku-TAN-e-us):   Pertaining to through the skin.

Percutaneous transhepatic cholangiography (per-ku-TAN-e-us trans-heh-PAT-ik kol-an-je-OG-rah-fe):   Bile vessels are imaged after injection of contrast material through the skin into the liver.

Perianal (per-e-A-nal):   Pertaining to surrounding the ANUS.

Periosteum (per-e-OS-te-um):   Membrane that surrounds bone.

Peritoneal (per-ih-to-NE-al):   Pertaining to the PERITONEUM.

Peritoneal dialysis (per-ih-to-NE-al di-AL-ih-sis):   Process of removing wastes from the blood by introducing a special fluid into the abdomen. The wastes pass into the fluid from the bloodstream, and then the fluid is drained from the body.

Peritoneoscopy (per-ih-to-ne-OS-ko-pe):   Visual examination of the peritoneal cavity with an endoscope. See LAPAROSCOPY.

Peritoneum (per-ih-to-NE-um):   Membrane that surrounds the abdomen and holds the abdominal organs in place.

Peritonitis (per-ih-to-NI-tis):   Inflammation of the peritoneum.

Phalanges (fah-LAN-jez):   Finger and toe bones.

Pharyngeal (fah-rin-JE-al):   Pertaining to the pharynx (throat).

Pharyngitis (fah-rin-JI-tis):   Inflammation of the pharynx (throat).

Pharynx (FAR-inks):   Organ behind the mouth that receives swallowed food and delivers it into the esophagus. The pharynx (throat) also receives air from the nose and passes it to the trachea (windpipe).

Phenothiazine (fe-no-THI-ah-zen):   Substance whose derivatives are used as tranquilizers and antipsychotic agents to treat mental illness.

Phlebitis (fleh-BI-tis):   Inflammation of a vein.

Phlebography (fle-BOG-ra-fe):   X-ray examination of veins after injection of contrast material.

Phlebotomy (fleh-BOT-o-me):   Incision of a vein.

Phrenic (FREH-nik):   Pertaining to the DIAPHRAGM.

Physical medicine and rehabilitation (FIZ-e-kal MED-i-sin and re-ha-bil-i-TA-shun):   Field of medicine that specializes in restoring the function of the body after illness.

Pineal gland (pi-NE-al gland):   Small endocrine gland within the brain that secretes the hormone melatonin, whose exact function is unclear. In lower animals the pineal gland is a receptor for light.

Pituitary gland (pih-TU-ih-tar-e gland):   Organ at the base of the brain that secretes hormones. These hormones enter the blood to regulate other organs and other endocrine glands.

Platelet (PLAT-let):   Cell in the blood that aids clotting; a thrombocyte.

Pleura (PLOO-rah):   Double membrane that surrounds the lungs. *Pleural* means pertaining to the pleura.

Pleural cavity (PLOO-ral KA-vih-te):   Space between the pleura surrounding the lungs.

Pleural effusion (PLOO-ral e-FU-zhun):   Collection of fluid between the double membrane surrounding the lungs.

Pleurisy (PLOO-rih-se):   Inflammation of the PLEURA.

Pleuritis (ploo-RI-tis):   Inflammation of the PLEURA.

Pneumoconiosis (noo-mo-ko-ne-O-sis):   Group of lung diseases resulting from inhalation of particles of dust such as coal, with permanent deposition of such particles in the lung.

Pneumonectomy (noo-mo-NEK-to-me):   Removal of a lung.

Pneumonia (noo-MO-ne-ah):   Abnormal condition of the lungs marked by inflammation and collection of material within the air sacs of the lungs.

Pneumonitis (noo-mo-NI-tis):   Inflammation of a lung or lungs.

Pneumothorax (noo-mo-THO-raks):   Abnormal accumulation of air in the space between the pleura.

Polycythemia (pol-e-si-THE-me-ah):   Increase in red blood cells. One form of polycythemia is polycythemia vera, in which the bone marrow produces an excess of erythrocytes and hemoglobin level is elevated.

Polydipsia (pol-e-DIP-se-ah):   Excessive thirst.

Polyneuropathy (pol-e-nu-ROP-ah-the):   Disease of many nerves.

Polyp (POL-ip):   A growth or mass (benign) protruding from a mucous membrane.

Polyuria (pol-e-UR-e-ah):   Excessive urination.

Postmortem (post-MOR-tem):   After death.

Postpartum (post-PAR-tum):   After birth.

Posterior (pos-TER-e-or):   Located in the back portion of a structure or of the body.

Precancerous (pre-KAN-ser-us):   Pertaining to a condition that may come before a cancer; a condition that tends to become malignant.

Prenatal (pre-NA-tal):   Pertaining to before birth.

Proctologist (prok-TOL-o-jist):   Physician who specializes in the study of the anus and rectum.

Proctoscopy (prok-TOS-ko-pe):   Inspection of the anus and rectum with a proctoscope (ENDOSCOPE). Proctoscopy is often performed before rectal surgery.

Proctosigmoidoscopy (prok-to-sig-moyd-OS-ko-pe):   Visual examination of the anus, rectum, and sigmoid colon with an endoscope.

Progesterone (pro-JES-teh-rone):   Hormone secreted by the ovaries to prepare to maintain the uterine lining during pregnancy.

Prognosis (prog-NO-sis):   Prediction as to the outcome of an illness or treatment. Prognosis literally means before (PRO-) knowledge (-GNOSIS).

Prolapse (pro-LAPS):   Falling down or drooping of a part of the body. Prolapse literally means sliding (-LAPSE) forward (PRO-).

Prostate gland (PROS-tat gland):   Male gland that surrounds the base of the urinary bladder. It produces fluid (semen) that leaves the body with sperm cells.

Prostatectomy (pros-tah-TEK-to-me):   Removal of the prostate gland.

Prostatic (pros-TAH-tik):   Pertaining to the prostate gland.

Prostatic carcinoma (pros-TAH-tik kar-si-NO-mah):   Malignant tumor arising from the PROSTATE GLAND. Also called *prostate cancer*.

Prostatic hyperplasia (pros-TAH-tik hi-per-PLA-zhah):   Abnormal increase in growth (benign) of the prostate gland.

Prosthesis (pros-THE-sis):   Artificial substitute for a missing part of the body. Prosthesis literally means to place (-THESIS) before (PROS-).

Proteinuria (pro-en-U-re-ah):   Abnormal condition of protein in the urine (albuminuria).

Psychiatrist (si-KI-ah-trist):   Specialist in the treatment of the mind and mental disorders.

Psychiatry (si-KI-ah-tre):   Treatment (IATR/O-) of disorders of the mind (PSYCH/O-).

Psychology (si-KOL-o-je):   Study of the mind, especially in relation to human behavior.

Psychosis (si-KO-sis):   Abnormal condition of the mind; a serious mental disorder that involves loss of normal perception of reality (pl. psychoses [si-KO-sez]).

Pulmonary (PUL-mo-ner-e):   Pertaining to the lungs.

Pulmonary circulation (PUL-mo-ner-e ser-ku-LA-shun):   Passage of blood from the heart to the lungs and back to the heart.

Pulmonary edema (PUL-mo-ner-e eh-DE-mah):   Abnormal collection of fluid in the lung (within the air sacs of the lung). Fluid backs up into lung tissue commonly due to congestive heart failure as the heart weakens and is unable to pump blood effectively.

Pulmonary embolism (PUL-mo-ner-e EM-bo-lizm):   Blockage of blood vessels by foreign matter (clot, tumor, fat, or air). The embolus frequently arises from the deep veins of the leg.

Pulmonary specialist (PUL-mo-ner-e SPESH-ah-list):   Physician trained to treat lung disorders.

Pupil (PU-pil):   Black center of the eye through which light enters.

Pyelitis (pi-eh-LI-tis):   Inflammation of the renal pelvis (central section of the kidney).

Pyelogram (PI-lo-gram):   Record of the renal pelvis after injection of contrast.

Q

Quadriplegia (kwad-ri-PLE-jah):   Paralysis of all four extremities and usually the trunk of the body caused by injury to the spinal cord in the cervical region of the spine.

R

Radiation oncologist (ra-de-A-shun ong-KOL-o-jist):   Physician trained in the treatment of disease (cancer) with high-energy x-rays or other particles.

Radiologist (ra-de-OL-o-jist):   Physician trained in the use of x-rays (including ultrasound and magnetic resonance imaging techniques) to diagnose illness.

Radiology (ra-de-OL-o-je):   Science of using x-rays in the diagnosis of disease.

Radiotherapy (ra-de-o-THER-ah-pe):   Treatment of disease (cancer) with high-energy particles such as x-rays and protons.

Radius (RA-de-us):   One of two lower arm bones. The radius is located on the thumb side of the hand.

Rectal resection (REK-tal re-SEK-shun):   Excision (resection) of the RECTUM.

Rectocele (REK-to-sel):   Hernia (protrusion) of the rectum into the vagina.

Rectum (REK-tum):   End of the colon. The rectum delivers wastes (feces) to the anus for elimination.

Relapse (re-LAPS):   Return of disease after its apparent termination.

Remission (re-MISH-un):   Lessening of symptoms of a disease.

Renal (RE-nal):   Pertaining to the kidney.

Renal failure (RE-nal FAL-ur):   Kidneys no longer function.

Renal pelvis (RE-nal PEL-vis):   Central section of the kidney, where urine collects.

Reproductive (re-pro-DUK-tiv):   Pertaining to the process by which living things produce offspring.

Research (RE-surch):   Laboratory investigation of a medical problem.

Resection (re-SEK-shun):   Removal (excision) of an organ or a structure.

Residency training (RES-i-den-se TRAY-ning):   Period of hospital work involving the care of patients after the completion of four years of medical school.

Respiratory system (RES-pir-ah-tor-e SIS-tem):   Organs that control breathing, allowing air to enter and leave the body.

Retina (RET-ih-nah):   Layer of sensitive cells at the back of the eye. Light is focused on the retina and then is transmitted to the optic nerve, which leads to the brain.

Retinopathy (reh-tih-NOP-ah-the):   Disease of the RETINA.

Retrogastric (reh-tro-GAS-trik):   Pertaining to behind the stomach.

Retroperitoneal (reh-tro-per-ih-to-NE-al):   Pertaining to behind the PERITONEUM.

Rhabdomyosarcoma (rab-do-mi-o-sar-KO-mah):   A malignant tumor of muscle cells (skeletal, voluntary muscle) that occurs most frequently in the head and neck, extremities, body wall, and area behind the abdomen.

Rheumatoid arthritis (ROO-mah-toyd arth-RI-tis):   Chronic inflammatory disease of the joints and connective tissue that leads to deformed joints.

Rheumatologist (roo-mah-TOL-o-jist):   Specialist in the treatment of diseases of connective tissues, especially the joints. RHEUMAT/O- comes from the Greek *rheuma,* meaning "that which flows, as a stream or a river." Inflammatory disorders of joints are often marked by a collection of fluid in joint spaces.

Rheumatology (roo-mah-TOL-o-je):   Branch of medicine dealing with inflammation, degeneration, or chemical changes in connective tissues, such as joints and muscles. Pain, stiffness, or limitation of motion are often characteristics of rheumatologic disorders.

Rhinitis (ri-NI-tis):   Inflammation of the nose.

Rhinoplasty (RI-no-plas-te):   Surgical repair of the nose.

Rhinorrhea (ri-no-RE-ah):   Discharge from the nose.

Rhinotomy (ri-NOT-o-me):   Incision of the nose.

Rib (rib):   One of twelve paired bones surrounding the chest. Seven ribs (true ribs) attach directly to the breastbone, three (false ribs) attach to the seventh rib, and two (floating ribs) are not attached at all.

S

Sacral (SA-kral):   Pertaining to the SACRUM.

Sacral region (SA-kral RE-jin):   Five fused bones in the lower back, below the lumbar bones and wedged between two parts of the hip (ilium).

Sacrum (SA-krum):   Triangular bone in the lower back, below the lumbar bones and formed by five fused bones.

Sagittal plane (SAJ-ih-tal plan):   An imaginary line that divides an organ or the body into right and left portions.

Sagittal section (SAJ-ih-tal SEK-shun):   Cut (section) through the body dividing it into a right and left portion.

Salpingectomy (sal-pin-JEK-to-me):   Removal of a fallopian (uterine) tube.

Salpingitis (sal-pin-JI-tis):   Inflammation of a fallopian (uterine) tube.

Sarcoidosis (sahr-koi-DO-sis):   Chronic, progressive disorder of cells in connective tissue, spleen, liver, bone marrow, lungs, and lymph nodes. Small collections of cells (granulomas) form in affected organs and tissues.

Sarcoma (sar-KO-mah):   Cancerous (malignant) tumor of connective tissue, such as bone, muscle, fat, or cartilage.

Scapula (SKAP-u-lah):   Shoulder bone.

Sclera (SKLE-rah):   White, outer coat of the eyeball.

Scrotal (SKRO-tal):   Pertaining to the scrotum.

Scrotum (SKRO-tum):   Sac on the outside of the body that contains the testes.

Sebaceous gland (seh-BA-shus gland):   Oil-producing (sebum-producing) gland in the skin.

Section (SEK-shun):   An act of cutting; a segment or subdivision of an organ.

Seizure (SE-zhur):   Convulsion (involuntary contraction of muscles) or attack of epilepsy. A seizure can also indicate a sudden attack or recurrence of a disease.

Sella turcica (SEL-ah TUR-sih-kah):   Cup-like depression at the base of the skull that holds the pituitary gland.

Semen (SE-men):   Fluid composed of sperm cells and secretions from the prostate gland and other male exocrine glands.

Seminoma (sem-ih-NO-mah):   Malignant tumor of the testis.

Sense organs (sens OR-ganz):   Parts of the body that receive messages from the environment and relay them to the brain so that we see, hear, and feel sensations. Examples of sense organs are the eye, the ear, and the skin.

Septic (SEP-tik):   Pertaining to infection.

Septicemia (sep-tih-SE-me-ah):   Infection in the blood. Septicemia is commonly called blood poisoning and is associated with the presence of bacteria or their poisons in the blood.

Shock (shok):   Group of symptoms (pale skin, rapid pulse, shallow breathing) that indicate poor oxygen supply to tissue and insufficient return of blood to the heart.

Sigmoid colon (SIG-moyd KO-len):   S-shaped lower portion of the colon.

Sigmoidoscopy (sig-moyd-OS-ko-pe):   Visual examination of the sigmoid colon with an endoscope inserted through the anus and rectum.

Sinus (SI-nus):   A cavity or space, such as in a bone. Also, refers to the sinoatrial node or pacemaker of the heart.

Skin (skin): Outer covering that protects the body.

Skull (skul): Bone that surrounds the brain and other organs in the head.

Small intestine (smal in-TES-tin): Organ that receives food from the stomach. The small intestine is divided into three sections: duodenum, jejunum, and ileum.

Sonogram (SON-o-gram): Record of sound waves after they bounce off organs in the body; an ULTRASOUND or echogram.

Spermatozoon (sper-mah-to-ZO-on): Sperm cell (pl. spermatozoa [sper-mah-to-ZO-ah]).

Spinal (SPI-nal): Pertaining to the spine (backbone).

Spinal cavity (SPI-nal KAV-ih-te): Space in the back that contains the spinal cord and is surrounded by the backbones.

Spinal column (SPI-nal KOL-um): Backbones; vertebrae.

Spinal cord (SPI-nal kord): Bundle of nerves that extends from the brain down the back. The spinal cord carries electrical messages to and from the spinal cord.

Spinal nerves (SPI-nal nervz): Nerves that transmit messages to and from the spinal cord.

Spleen (splen): Organ in the left upper quadrant of the abdomen. The spleen stores blood cells and destroys red blood cells while producing white blood cells called LYMPHOCYTES.

Splenectomy (splehn-EK-to-me): Removal of the spleen.

Splenomegaly (splehn-o-MEG-ah-le): Enlargement of the spleen.

Spondylitis (spon-dih-LI-tis): Chronic, serious inflammatory disorder of backbones involving erosion and collapse of vertebrae. See ANKYLOSING SPONDYLITIS.

Spondylosis (spon-dih-LO-sis): Abnormal condition of a vertebra or vertebrae.

Sputum (SPU-tum): Material expelled from the lungs and expelled through the mouth.

Sternum (STER-num): Breast bone.

Stomach (STUM-ak): Organ that receives food from the esophagus and sends it to the small intestine. Enzymes in the stomach break down food particles during digestion.

Stomatitis (sto-mah-TI-tis): Inflammation of the mouth.

Stroke (strok): Trauma to or blockage of blood vessels within the brain, leading to a reduction in the blood supply to brain tissue. This causes nerve cells in the brain to die and results in loss of function to the part of the body controlled by those nerve cells.

Subcostal (sub-KOS-tal): Pertaining to below the ribs.

Subcutaneous tissue (sub-ku-TA-ne-us TIS-u): Lower layer of the skin composed of fatty tissue.

Subdural hematoma (sub-DUR-al he-mah-TO-mah): Collection of blood under the dura mater (outermost layer of the membranes surrounding the brain).

Subgastric (sub-GAS-trik): Pertaining to below the stomach.

Subhepatic (sub-heh-PAT-ik): Pertaining to under the liver.

Subscapular (sub-SKAP-u-lar): Pertaining to under the shoulder bone.

Subtotal (sub-TO-tal): Less than total; just under the total amount.

Suprarenal glands (soo-prah-RE-nal glanz): Two endocrine glands, each located above a kidney. Also called adrenal glands.

Surgery (SUR-jer-e): Branch of medicine that treats disease by manual (hand) or operative methods.

Sweat gland (sweht gland): Organ in the skin that produces a watery substance containing salts.

Syncope (SING-kah-pe): Fainting; sudden loss of consciousness.

Syndrome (SIN-drom):   Set of symptoms and signs of disease that occur together to indicate a disease condition.

System (SIS-tem):   Group of organs working together to do a job in the body. For example, the digestive system includes the mouth, throat, stomach, and intestines, all of which help to bring food into the body, break it down, and deliver it to the bloodstream.

Systemic circulation (sis-TEM-ik ser-ku-LA-shun):   Passage of blood from the heart to the tissues of the body and back to the heart.

Systemic lupus erythematosus (sis-TEM-ik LOO-pus er-ih-the-mah-TO-SUS):   Chronic inflammatory disease affecting many systems of the body (joints, skin, kidneys, and nerves). A red (erythematous) rash over the nose and cheeks is characteristic.

T

Tachycardia (tak-eh-KAR-de-ah):   Condition of fast, rapid heartbeat.

Tachypnea (tak-ip-NE-ah):   Condition of rapid breathing.

Tendinitis (ten-dih-NI-tis):   Inflammation of a tendon.

Tendon (TEN-don):   Connective tissue that joins muscles to bones.

Tenorrhaphy (ten-OR-ah-fe):   Suture of a tendon.

Testicle (TES-tih-kl):   See TESTIS.

Testicular carcinoma (tes-TIK-u-lar kar-sih-NO-mah):   Malignant tumor originating in a testis. An example is a SEMINOMA.

Testis (TES-tis):   One of two paired male organs in the scrotal sac. The testes (pl.) produce sperm cells and male hormone (testosterone). Also called a testicle.

Testosterone (tes-TOS-teh-ron):   A hormone that produces male secondary sex characteristics; an ANDROGEN.

Thoracentesis (tho-rah-sen-TE-sis):   Surgical puncture of the chest to remove fluid; thoracocentesis.

Thoracic (tho-RAS-ik):   Pertaining to the chest.

Thoracic cavity (tho-RAS-ik KAV-ih-te):   Space above the abdomen that contains the heart, lungs, and other organs; the chest cavity.

Thoracic region (tho-RAS-ik RE-jin):   Backbones attached to the ribs and located in the region of the chest, between the neck and the waist.

Thoracic surgeon (tho-RAS-ik SUR-jin):   Physician who operates on organs in the chest.

Thoracic vertebra (tho-RAS-ik VER-teh-brah):   A backbone in the region of the chest.

Thoracotomy (tho-rah-KOT-o-me):   Incision of the chest.

Throat (throt):   See PHARYNX.

Thrombocyte (THROM-bo-sit):   Clotting cell; a platelet.

Thrombolytic therapy (throm-bo-LIT-ik THER-ah-pe):   Treatment with drugs such as streptokinase and tPA (tissue plasminogen activator) to dissolve clots that may cause a heart attack.

Thrombophlebitis (throm-bo-fle-BI-tis):   Inflammation of a vein accompanied by formation of a clot.

Thrombosis (throm-BO-sis):   Abnormal condition of clot formation.

Thrombus (THROM-bus):   Blood clot.

Thymoma (thi-MO-mah):   Tumor (malignant) of the thymus gland.

Thymus gland (THI-mus gland):   Endocrine gland in the middle of the chest that produces the hormone *thymosin*. A much larger gland in children, the thymus aids the immune system by stimulating the production of white blood cells (lymphocytes).

Thyroadenitis (thi-ro-ah-deh-NI-tis):   Inflammation of the thyroid gland.

Thyroidectomy (thi-roy-DEK-to-me):   Removal of the thyroid gland.

Thyroid gland (THI-royd gland):   Endocrine gland in the neck that produces hormones, which act on cells all over the body. The hormones increase the activity of cells by stimulating metabolism and the release of energy.

Thyroid-stimulating hormone (THI-royd STIM-ula-ting HOR-mon):   Hormone secreted by the pituitary gland to stimulate the thyroid gland to produce its hormones, such as thyroxine. Also called TSH.

Thyroxine (thi-ROK-sin):   Hormone secreted by the thyroid gland. Also known as T_4.

Tibia (TIB-e-ah):   Larger of the two lower leg bones; the shin bone.

Tinnitus (TIN-ih-tus):   Noise in the ears, such as ringing, roaring, or buzzing.

Tissue (TISH-u):   Groups of similar cells that work together to do a job in the body. Examples are muscle tissue, nerve tissue, and epithelial (skin) tissue.

Tissue capillaries (TISH-u KAP-ih-lar-ez):   Tiny blood vessels that lie near cells and through whose walls gases, food, and waste materials pass.

Tomography (to-MOG-rah-fe):   Series of x-ray images that show an organ in depth by producing images of single tissue planes.

Tonsillectomy (ton-sih-LEK-to-me):   Removal (excision) of a tonsil or TONSILS.

Tonsillitis (ton-sih-LI-tis):   Inflammation of the TONSILS.

Tonsils (TON-silz):   Lymphatic tissue in the back of the mouth near the throat.

Trachea (TRAY-ke-ah):   Tube that carries air from the throat to the BRONCHIAL TUBES; the windpipe.

Tracheitis (tray-ke-I-tis):   Inflammation of the trachea.

Tracheostomy (tray-ke-OS-to-me):   Opening of the trachea to the outside of the body.

Tracheotomy (tray-ke-OT-o-me):   Incision of the trachea.

Transabdominal (trans-ab-DOM-ih-nal):   Pertaining to across the abdomen.

Transdermal (tranz-DER-mal):   Pertaining to through the skin.

Transgastric (trans-GAS-trik):   Pertaining to across (through) the stomach.

Transhepatic (tranz-he-PAH-tik):   Pertaining to across or through the liver.

Transurethral (trans-u-RE-thral):   Pertaining to across (through) the urethra. A TURP is a transurethral resection of the prostate by surgery through the urethra.

Transvaginal ultrasound (tranz-VAH-jin-al UL-trah-sound):   A sound probe is placed in the vagina and ultrasound images are made of the pelvic organs (uterus and ovaries).

Transverse plane (trans-VERS plan):   Imaginary line that divides an organ or the body into an upper and lower portion; a cross-sectional view.

Tricuspid valve (tri-KUS-pid valv):   Fold of tissue between the upper and lower chambers on the right side of the heart. It has three cusps or points and prevents backflow of blood into the right ATRIUM when the heart is pumping blood.

Triglyceride (tri-GLIS-eh-ride):   Fat consisting of three molecules of fatty acid and glycerol. It makes up most animal and vegetable fats and is the major lipid (fat) in blood.

Tuberculosis (too-ber-ku-LO-sis):   Infectious, inflammatory disease that commonly affects the lungs, although it can occur in any part of the body. It is caused by the tubercle bacillus (type of bacteria).

Tympanic membrane (tim-PAN-ik MEM-bran):   See EARDRUM.
Tympanoplasty (tim-pan-o-PLAS-te):   Surgical repair of the eardrum.

U

Ulcer (UL-ser):   Sore or defect in the surface of an organ. Ulcers are produced by destruction of tissue.
Ulcerative colitis (UL-seh-rah-tiv ko-LI-tis):   Recurrent inflammatory disorder marked by ulcers in the large bowel. Along with Crohn disease, ulcerative colitis is an INFLAMMATORY BOWEL DISEASE.
Ulna (UL-nah):   One of two lower arm bones. The ulna is located on the little finger side of the hand.
Ultrasonography (ul-trah-so-NOG-rah-fe):   Recording of internal body structures with sound waves.
Ultrasound (UL-tra-sownd):   Sound waves with greater frequency than can be heard by the human ear. This energy is used to detect abnormalities by beaming the waves into the body and recording echoes that reflect off tissues.
Unilateral (u-nih-LAT-er-al):   Pertaining to one side.
Upper gastrointestinal (GI) series (UP-per gas-tro-in-TES-tin-al SER-ez):   Barium is swallowed and x-ray images are taken of the esophagus, stomach, and small intestine.
Urea (u-RE-ah):   Chief nitrogen-containing waste that the kidney removes from the blood and eliminates from the body in urine.
Uremia (u-RE-me-ah):   Abnormal condition of excessive amounts of urea in the bloodstream.
Ureter (YOOR-eh-ter or u-RE-ter):   One of two tubes that lead from the kidney to the urinary bladder.
Ureterectomy (u-re-ter-EK-to-me):   Removal (excision) of a ureter.
Urethra (u-RE-thrah):   Tube that carries urine from the urinary bladder to the outside of the body. In males, the urethra, which is within the penis, also carries sperm from the VANS DEFERENS to the outside of the body when sperm are discharged (ejaculation).
Urethral stricture (u-RE-thral STRIK-shur):   Narrowing of the urethra.
Urethritis (u-re-THRI-tis):   Inflammation of the urethra.
Urinalysis (u-rih-NAL-ih-sis):   Examination of urine to determine its contents.
Urinary bladder (UR-in-er-e BLA-der):   Muscular sac that holds urine and then releases it to leave the body through the urethra.
Urinary catheterization (UR-in-er-e kath-eh-ter-ih-ZA-shun):   Catheter (tube) is passed through the urethra into the urinary bladder for short-term or long-term drainage of urine.
Urinary system (UR-in-er-e SIS-tem):   Organs that produce and send urine out of the body. These organs are the kidneys, ureters, bladder, and urethra.
Urinary tract (UR-in-er-e trakt):   Tubes and organs that carry urine from the kidney to the outside of the body.
Urine (UR-in):   Fluid that is produced by the kidneys, passed through the ureters, stored in the bladder, and released from the body through the urethra.
Urologist (u-ROL-o-jist):   Specialist in operating on the urinary tract in males and females and on the reproductive tract in males.

Urology (u-ROL-o-je):   Study of the urinary system in males and females and the reproductive tract in males.

Uterine (U-ter-in):   Pertaining to the uterus.

Uterine tubes (U-ter-in tubz):   See FALLOPIAN TUBES.

Uterus (U-ter-us):   Muscular organ in a female that holds and provides nourishment for the developing fetus; the WOMB.

$\mathcal{V}$

Vagina (vah-JI-nah):   Muscular passageway from the uterus to the outside of the body.

Vaginitis (vah-jih-NI-tis):   Inflammation of the vagina.

Varicocele (VAR-ih-ko-sel):   Swollen, twisted veins within the spermatic cord, above the testes. It produces a swelling in the scrotum that feels like a "bag of worms."

Varix (VAH-riks):   Enlarged, swollen, tortuous veins (pl. varices [VAH-ri-sez]).

Vas deferens (vas DEHF-or-enz):   One of two tubes that carry sperm from the testes to the urethra for ejaculation.

Vascular (VAS-ku-lar):   Pertaining to blood vessels.

Vasculitis (vas-ku-LI-tis):   Inflammation of blood vessels.

Vasectomy (vas-EK-to-me):   Removal of the vas deferens or a portion of it so that sperm cells are prevented from becoming part of SEMEN.

Vasoconstrictor (vas-o-kon-STRIK-tor):   Drug that narrows blood vessels, especially small arteries.

Vasodilator (vas-o-DI-la-tor):   Agent that widens blood vessels.

Vein (van):   Blood vessel that carries blood back to the heart from tissues of the body.

Ventricle (VEN-tri-kl):   One of the two lower chambers of the heart. The right ventricle receives blood from the right atrium (upper chamber) and sends it to the lungs. The left ventricle receives blood from the left atrium and sends it to the body through the aorta.

Venule (VEN-ul):   Small vein.

Venulitis (ven-u-LI-tis):   Inflammation of a small vein.

Vertebra (VER-teh-brah):   A backbone.

Vertebrae (VER-teh-bray):   Backbones.

Vertebral (VER-teh-bral):   Pertaining to a backbone.

Vesical (VES-ih-kal):   Pertaining to the urinary bladder (VESIC/O-).

Virus (VI-rus):   Small infectious agent that can reproduce itself only when it is inside another living cell (host).

Visceral (VIS-er-al):   Pertaining to internal organs.

$\mathcal{W}$

Womb (woom):   See UTERUS.

Glossary
of Word Parts

Section I of this glossary is a list of **medical terminology** word parts and their **English** meanings. Section II is the reverse of that list, giving **English** meanings and their corresponding **medical terminology** word parts. If you wish to identify various combining forms, suffixes, and prefixes for the corresponding English term, check Section II.

SECTION I: MEDICAL TERMINOLOGY → ENGLISH

Word Part	Meaning
a-, an-	no, not
ab-	away from
abdomin/o	abdomen
-ac	pertaining to
ad-	toward
aden/o	gland
adenoid/o	adenoids
adren/o	adrenal gland
-al	pertaining to
-algia	pain
alveol/o	alveolus (air sac within the lung)
amni/o	amnion (sac that surrounds the embryo)
-an	pertaining to
ana-	up, apart
an/o	anus
angi/o	vessel (blood)
ante-	before, forward
anter/o	front
anti-	against
aort/o	aorta
append/o, appendic/o	appendix
-ar	pertaining to
arteri/o	artery
arteriol/o	small artery
arthr/o	joint
-ary	pertaining to
ather/o	fatty plaque
-ation	process, condition
aur/o	ear
aut-	self
axill/o	armpit
balan/o	penis
bi-	two
bi/o	life

blephar/o	eyelid
brady-	slow
bronch/o	bronchial tube
bronchiol/o	small bronchial tube
calcane/o	calcaneus (heel bone)
capillar/o	capillary
carcin/o	cancer, cancerous
cardi/o	heart
carp/o	wrist bones (carpals)
-cele	hernia
-centesis	surgical puncture to remove fluid
cephal/o	head
cerebell/o	cerebellum (posterior part of the brain)
cerebr/o	cerebrum (largest part of the brain)
cervic/o	neck
chem/o	drug, chemical
cholecyst/o	gallbladder
choledoch/o	common bile duct
chondr/o	cartilage
chron/o	time
-cision	process of cutting
cis/o	to cut
clavicul/o	clavicle (collar bone)
-coccus	bacterium (berry-shaped); pl. -cocci
coccyg/o	tailbone
col/o	colon (large intestine)
colon/o	colon
colp/o	vagina
comi/o	to care for
con-	with, together
coni/o	dust
-coniosis	abnormal condition of dust
coron/o	heart
cost/o	rib
crani/o	skull
crin/o	secrete
-crine	secretion
-crit	separation
cry/o	cold
cutane/o	skin
cyan/o	blue
cyst/o	urinary bladder
cyt/o	cell
-cyte	cell

dactyl/o	fingers or toes
dermat/o, derm/o	skin
dia-	thorough, complete
-dipsia	thirst
duoden/o	duodenum
dur/o	dura mater (outermost meningeal layer)
-dynia	pain
dys-	abnormal, bad, difficult, painful
-eal	pertaining to
ec-	out, outside
-ectasia, -ectasis	dilation, stretching, widening
ecto-	out, outside
-ectomy	excision (resection, removal); process of cutting out
electr/o	electricity
-emesis	vomiting
-emia	blood condition
en-	within, in, inner
encephal/o	brain
endo-	within, in, inner
endocrin/o	endocrine glands
endometr/o, endometri/o	endometrium (inner lining of the uterus)
enter/o	intestines (usually small intestine)
epi-	above, upon
epiglott/o	epiglottis
epitheli/o	skin (surface tissue)
erythr/o	red
esophag/o	esophagus
esthesi/o	sensation
ex-, exo-, extra-	out, outside
femor/o	femur, thigh bone
fibr/o	fibrous tissue
fibul/o	fibula (smaller lower leg bone)
gastr/o	stomach
gen/o	to produce
-gen	to produce
-genesis	producing, forming
-genic	pertaining to producing, produced by
ger/o	old age
glyc/o	sugar
gnos/o	knowledge
-gram	record
-graph	instrument to record
-graphy	process of recording, to record
gynec/o	woman, female

hemat/o, hem/o	blood
hepat/o	liver
humer/o	humerus (upper arm bone)
hydr/o	water
hyper-	above, excessive, more than normal, too much
hypo-	below, deficient, less than normal, too little
hypophys/o	pituitary gland
hyster/o	uterus
-ia	condition
-ian	practitioner
iatr/o	treatment
-ic	pertaining to
ile/o	ileum (third part of small intestine)
ili/o	ilium (upper part of hip bone)
in-	in, into
-ine	pertaining to
infra-	below
inguin/o	groin
inter-	between
intra-	within
-ior	pertaining to
isch/o	to hold back
-ism	condition, process
-ist	specialist
-itis	inflammation
jejun/o	jejunum
lapar/o	abdomen
-lapse	slide
laryng/o	larynx (voice box)
later/o	side
ligament/o	ligament
leiomy/o	smooth muscle
leuk/o	white
lip/o	fat
-listhesis	to slip, slide
lith/o	stone
-lith	stone
-logy	study of, process of study
lumb/o	loin, waist region
lymph/o	lymph
lymphaden/o	lymph nodes
lymphangi/o	lymph vessel
lys/o	separation, breakdown, destruction
-lysis	separation, breakdown, destruction

mal-	bad
-malacia	softening
mamm/o	breast
mast/o	breast
mediastin/o	mediastinum
medull/o	medulla oblongata (lower part of the brain)
-megaly	enlargement
men/o	menstruation
mening/o	meninges (membranes covering brain and spinal cord)
meta-	beyond, change
metacarp/o	metacarpals (hand bones)
metatars/o	metatarsals (foot bones)
-meter	to measure
metr/o, metri/o	uterus; to measure
-metry	measurement
-mortem	death
-motor	movement
muscul/o	muscle
my/o	muscle
myel/o	bone marrow (with -blast, -oma, -cyte, -genous)
myel/o	spinal cord (with -gram, -itis, -cele)
myos/o	muscle
myring/o	eardrum
nas/o	nose
nat/i	birth
necr/o	death
neo-	new
nephr/o	kidney
neur/o	nerve
norm/o	rule, order
nos/o	disease
obstetr/o	midwife
ocul/o	eye
-oid	pertaining to, resembling
-oma	tumor, mass, swelling
onc/o	tumor
o/o	egg
oophor/o	ovary
ophthalm/o	eye
-opsy	process of viewing
opt/o, optic/o	eye
or/o	mouth
orch/o	testicle, testis
orchi/o	testicle, testis

orchid/o	testicle, testis
orth/o	straight
-osis	abnormal condition
osm/o	smell
oste/o	bone
ot/o	ear
-ous	pertaining to
ovari/o	ovary
pancreat/o	pancreas
para-	beside, near, along the side of
parathyroid/o	parathyroid gland
-partum	birth
path/o	disease
-pathy	disease condition
ped/o	child
pelv/o	hip bone
-penia	deficiency
per-	through
peri-	surrounding
peritone/o	peritoneum (membrane around abdominal organs)
perone/o	fibula
-pexy	fixation (surgical)
phak/o	lens of the eye
phalang/o	phalanges (finger and toe bones)
pharyng/o	pharynx, throat
-phasia	speech
-philia	attraction to
phleb/o	vein
phren/o	diaphragm
phren/o	mind
pituitar/o	pituitary gland
plas/o	formation, growth, development
-plasm	formation, growth, development
-plasia	formation, growth
-plasty	surgical repair
-plegia	paralysis
pleur/o	pleura (membranes surrounding the lungs)
-pnea	breathing
pneum/o	air, lung
pneumon/o	lung
-poiesis	formation
poly-	many, much
post-	after, behind
poster/o	back, behind
pre-	before

pro-, pros-	before, forward
proct/o	anus and rectum
prostat/o	prostate gland
psych/o	mind
-ptosis	prolapse, sagging
-ptysis	spitting
pulmon/o	lung
pyel/o	renal pelvis (central section of the kidney)
radi/o	x-ray; radius (lateral lower arm bone)
re-, retro-	behind, back
rect/o	rectum
ren/o	kidney
retin/o	retina of the eye
rhabdomy/o	striated (skeletal) muscle
rheumat/o	flow, fluid
rhin/o	nose
-rrhage	bursting forth of blood
-rrhagia	bursting forth of blood
-rrhaphy	suture
-rrhea	flow, discharge
sacr/o	sacrum
salping/o	fallopian (uterine) tube; eustachian tube
-salpinx	fallopian (uterine) tube; eustachian tube
sarc/o	flesh
scapul/o	shoulder blade (bone)
-sclerosis	hardening
-scope	instrument to view or visually examine
-scopy	process of viewing or visual examination
scrot/o	scrotal sac, scrotum
-section	to cut
sept/o	infection
septic/o	infection
-sis	condition
-somatic	pertaining to the body
son/o	sound
-spasm	constriction
spin/o	backbone, spine, vertebra
splen/o	spleen
spondyl/o	vertebra, backbone
-stasis	stop, control; place, to stand
-stat	stop, control
-stenosis	narrowing
stern/o	sternum (breast bone)
stomat/o	mouth
-stomy	opening

sub-	under, below
sym-	with, together (use before b, p, and m)
syn-	with, together
tachy-	fast
tendin/o, ten/o	tendon
-tension	pressure
theli/o, thel/o	nipple
-therapy	treatment
-thesis	to put, to place
thorac/o	chest
thromb/o	clot
thym/o	thymus gland
thyr/o, thyroid/o, thyroaden/o	thyroid gland
tibi/o	tibia or shin bone (larger lower leg bone)
-tic	pertaining to
-tomy	incision, process of cutting into
tonsill/o	tonsils
top/o	to put, place
trache/o	trachea, windpipe
trans-	across, through
tri-	three
troph/o	development, nourishment
-trophy	development, nourishment
tympan/o	eardrum
uln/o	ulna (medial lower arm bone)
ultra-	beyond
-um	structure
uni-	one
ureter/o	ureter
urethr/o	urethra
ur/o	urine, urinary tract
-uria	urine condition
uter/o	uterus
vagin/o	vagina
vas/o	vessel, vas deferens
vascul/o	blood vessel
ven/o	vein
venul/o	venule
vertebr/o	vertebra, backbone
vesic/o	urinary bladder
-y	condition, process

SECTION II: ENGLISH → MEDICAL TERMINOLOGY

Meaning	Word Part
abdomen	abdomin/o (use with -al, -centesis)
	lapar/o (use with -scope, -scopy, -tomy)
abnormal	dys-
abnormal condition	-osis
abnormal condition of dust	-coniosis
above	epi-, hyper-
across	trans-
adenoids	adenoid/o
adrenal gland	adren/o
after	post-
against	anti-
air	pneum/o
air sac	alveol/o
along the side of	para-
alveolus	alveol/o
amnion	amni/o
anus	an/o
anus and rectum	proct/o
aorta	aort/o
apart	ana-
appendix	append/o (use with -ectomy)
	appendic/o (use with -itis)
armpit	axill/o
artery	arteri/o
attraction to	-philia
away from	ab-
back	poster/o, re-, retro-
backbone	spin/o (use with -al)
	spondyl/o (use with -itis, -listhesis, -osis, -pathy)
	vertebr/o (use with -al)
bacterium (berry-shaped)	-coccus (pl. -cocci)
bad	dys-, mal-
before	ante-, pre-, pro-, pros-
behind	post-, poster/o, re-, retro-
below	hypo-, infra-, sub-
beside	para-
between	inter-
beyond	meta-, ultra-
birth	nat/i, -partum

bladder (urinary)	cyst/o (use with -ic, -itis, -cele, -gram, -scopy)
	vesic/o (use with -al, -stomy, -tomy)
blood	hem/o (use with -cyte, -dialysis, -globin, -lysis, -philia, -ptysis, -rrhage, -stasis, -stat)
	hemat/o (use with -crit, -emesis, -logist, -logy, -oma, -poiesis, -salpinx, -uria)
blood condition	-emia
blood vessel	angi/o (use with -ectomy, -dysplasia, -genesis, -gram, -graphy, -oma, -plasty, -spasm)
	vas/o (use with -constriction, -dilatation, -motor)
	vascul/o (use with -ar, -itis)
blue	cyan/o
body	-somatic
bone	oste/o
bone marrow	myel/o
brain	encephal/o
breakdown	-lysis, lys/o
breast	mamm/o (use with -ary, -gram, -graphy, -plasty)
	mast/o (use with -algia, -ectomy, -itis)
breast bone	stern/o
breathing	-pnea
bronchial tube	bronch/o
bronchiole	bronchiol/o
bursting forth of blood	-rrhage, -rrhagia
calcaneus	calcane/o
cancer	carcin/o
cancerous	carcin/o
capillary	capillar/o
care for (to)	comi/o
carpals	carp/o
cartilage	chondr/o
cell	-cyte, cyt/o
cerebellum	cerebell/o
cerebrum	cerebr/o
change	meta-
chemical	chem/o
chest	thorac/o
child	ped/o
clavicle	clavicul/o
clot	thromb/o
cold	cry/o
collarbone	clavicul/o
colon	col/o (use with -ectomy, -itis, -stomy)
	colon/o (use with -pathy, -scope, -scopy)
common bile duct	choledoch/o

complete	dia-
condition	-ation, -ia, -ism, -osis, -sis, -y
condition of blood	-emia
constriction	-spasm
control	-stasis, -stat
cut	-cision, cis/o, -section, -tomy
death	-mortem, necr/o
deficiency	-penia
deficient	hypo-
destruction	lys/o, -lysis
development	troph/o, -trophy, plas/o, -plasm
dilation	-ectasia, -ectasis
diaphragm	phren/o
difficult	dys-
discharge	-rrhea
disease	path/o, -pathy; nos/o
drug	chem/o
duodenum	duoden/o
dura mater	dur/o
dust	coni/o
dust condition	-coniosis
ear	ot/o, aur/o
eardrum	myring/o (use with -ectomy, -itis, -tomy)
	tympan/o (use with -ic, -metry, -plasty)
egg	o/o
electricity	electr/o
endocrine gland	endocrin/o
endometrium	endometri/o
enlargement	-megaly
epiglottis	epiglott/o
esophagus	esophag/o
eustachian tube	salping/o, -salpinx
excessive	hyper-
excision	-ectomy
eye	ocul/o (use with -ar, -facial, -motor)
	ophthalm/o (use with -ia, -ic, -logist, -logy, -pathy, -plasty, -plegia, -scope, -scopy)
	opt/o (use with -ic, -metrist)
	optic/o (use with -ian)
eyelid	blephar/o
fallopian tube	salping/o, -salpinx
fast	tachy-
fat	lip/o

fatty plaque	ather/o
female	gynec/o
femur	femor/o
fibrous tissue	fibr/o
fibula	fibul/o, perone/o
fingers	dactyl/o
fixation (surgical)	-pexy
flesh	sarc/o
flow	-rrhea, rheumat/o
fluid	rheumat/o
foot bones	metatars/o
formation	-plasia, plas/o, -plasm, -poiesis, -genesis
forward	ante-, pro-, pros-
front	anter/o
gallbladder	cholecyst/o
gland	aden/o
groin	inguin/o
growth	plas/o, -plasm
hand bones	metacarp/o
hardening	-sclerosis
head	cephal/o
heart	cardi/o (use with -ac, -graphy, -logy, -logist, -megaly, -pathy, -vascular)
	coron/o (use with -ary)
heel bone	calcane/o
hernia	-cele
hip bone	pelv/o
hold back (to)	isch/o
humerus	humer/o
ileum	ile/o
ilium	ili/o
in, into	in-, en-, endo-
incision	-tomy, -section
infection	sept/o, septic/o
inflammation	-itis
inner	en-, endo-
instrument to record	-graph
instrument to view	-scope
intestines (small)	enter/o
jejunum	jejun/o
joint	arthr/o

kidney	nephr/o (use with -algia, -ectomy, -ic, -itis, -lith, -megaly, -oma, -osis, -pathy, -ptosis, -sclerosis, -stomy, -tomy)
	ren/o (use with -al, -gram)
kidney (central section)	pyel/o
knowledge	gnos/o
larynx	laryng/o
lens of the eye	phak/o
less than normal	hypo-
life	bi/o
ligament	ligament/o
liver	hepat/o
loin	lumb/o
lung	pneum/o (use with -coccus, -coniosis, -thorax)
	pneumon/o (use with -ectomy, -ia, -ic, -itis, -pathy)
	pulmon/o (use with -ary)
lymph	lymph/o
lymph node	lymphaden/o
lymph vessel	lymphangi/o
mass	-oma
many	poly-
measure (to)	metr/o, -meter, -metry
mediastinum	mediastin/o
medulla oblongata	medull/o
meninges	mening/o
menstruation	men/o
metacarpals	metacarp/o
metatarsals	metatars/o
midwife	obstetr/o
mind	psych/o, phren/o
more than normal	hyper-
mouth	or/o (use with -al)
	stomat/o (use with -itis)
movement	-motor
much	poly-
muscle	muscul/o (use with -ar, -skeletal)
	myos/o (use with -itis)
	my/o (use with -algia, -ectomy, -oma, -gram, -neural)
narrowing	-stenosis
near	para-
neck	cervic/o
nerve	neur/o
new	neo-
nipple	theli/o, thel/o

no, not	a-, an-
nose	nas/o (use with -al)
	rhin/o (use with -itis, -rrhea, -plasty)
nourishment	troph/o, -trophy
old age	ger/o
one	uni-
opening	-stomy
order	norm/o
out, outside	ec-, ecto-, ex-, exo- extra-
ovary	oophor/o (use with -itis, -ectomy, -pexy, -plasty, -tomy)
	ovari/o (use with -an)
pain	-algia, -dynia
painful	dys-
pancreas	pancreat/o
paralysis	-plegia
parathyroid gland	parathyroid/o
pelvis	pelv/o
pelvis (renal)	pyel/o
penis	balan/o
peritoneum	peritone/o
pertaining to	-ac, -al, -an, -ar, -ary, -eal, -ic, -ine, -ior, -oid, -ous, -tic
pertaining to the body	-somatic
phalanges	phalang/o
pharynx	pharyng/o
pituitary gland	hypophys/o, pituitar/o
place	top/o, -stasis
pleura	pleur/o
practitioner	-ian
pressure	-tension
process	-ation, -ism, -y
process of cutting into	-cision, -tomy, -section
process of cutting out	-ectomy
process of recording	-graphy
process of viewing	-opsy, -scopy
produce (to)	-gen, gen/o
produced by	-genic
producing	-genic, -genesis
prolapse	-ptosis
prostate gland	prostat/o
puncture to remove fluid	-centesis
put, place (to)	top/o, -thesis
radius (lower arm bone)	radi/o

record	-gram
recording (process)	-graphy
rectum	rect/o
red	erythr/o
removal	-ectomy
renal pelvis	pyel/o
repair	-plasty
resection	-ectomy
resembling	-oid
retina of the eye	retin/o
rib	cost/o
rule	norm/o
sacrum	sacr/o
sagging	-ptosis
scapula	scapul/o
scrotum, scrotal sac	scrot/o
secrete, secretion	-crine, crin/o
self	aut-
sensation	esthesi/o
separation	-crit, -lysis, lys/o
shin bone	tibi/o
shoulder blade	scapul/o
side	later/o
skin	cutane/o (use with -ous)
	derm/o (use with -al); dermat/o (use with -itis, -logy, -osis)
	epitheli/o (use with -al)
skull	crani/o
slide	-lapse, -listhesis
slip (to)	-listhesis
slow	brady-
small artery	arteriol/o
small bronchial tube	bronchiol/o
small intestine	enter/o
smell	osm/o
smooth muscle	leiomy/o
softening	-malacia
sound	son/o
specialist	-ist
speech	-phasia
spinal cord	myel/o
spine	spin/o
spitting	-ptysis
spleen	splen/o
stand (to)	-stasis

sternum	stern/o
stomach	gastr/o
stone	lith/o, -lith
stop	-stasis, -stat
straight	orth/o
stretching	-ectasia, -ectasis
striated (skeletal) muscle	rhabdomy/o
structure	-um
study of	-logy
sugar	glyc/o
surgical puncture to remove fluid	-centesis
surgical repair	-plasty
surrounding	peri-
suture	-rrhaphy
swelling	-oma
tailbone	coccyg/o
tendon	tendin/o, ten/o
testicle, testis	orch/o, orchi/o, orchid/o
thigh bone	femor/o
thirst	-dipsia
throat	pharyng/o
three	tri-
through	dia-, per-, trans-
thymus gland	thym/o
thyroid gland	thyr/o, thyroid/o, thyroaden/o
tibia	tibi/o
time	chron/o
toes	dactyl/o
together	con-, syn-, sym-
tonsil	tonsill/o
too much	hyper-
too little	hypo-
toward	ad-
trachea	trache/o
treatment	iatr/o, -therapy
tumor	-oma, onc/o
two	bi-
ulna	uln/o
under	hypo-, sub-
up	ana-
upon	epi-
ureter	ureter/o

urethra	urethr/o
urinary bladder	cyst/o, vesic/o
urinary tract	ur/o
urine	ur/o
urine condition	-uria
uterus	hyster/o (use with -ectomy, -graphy, -gram)
	metr/o (use with -itis, -rrhagia)
	metri/o (use with -al)
	uter/o (use with -ine)
uterus (inner lining)	endometr/o, endometri/o
vagina	colp/o (use with -pexy, -plasty, -scope, -scopy, -tomy)
	vagin/o (use with -al, -itis)
vas deferens	vas/o
vein	phleb/o (use with -ectomy, -itis, -lith, -thrombosis, -tomy)
	ven/o (use with -ous, -gram)
venule	venul/o
vertebra	spin/o (use with -al)
	spondyl/o (use with -itis, -listhesis, -osis, -pathy)
	vertebr/o (use with -al)
vessel	angi/o (use with -ectomy, -dysplasia, -genesis, -gram, -graphy, -oma, -plasty, -spasm)
	vas/o (use with -constriction, -dilation, -motor)
	vascul/o (use with -ar, -itis)
view (to)	-opsy
visual examination	-scopy
voice box	laryng/o
vomiting	-emesis
waist region	lumb/o
water	hydr/o
white	leuk/o
widening	-ectasia, -ectasis
windpipe	trache/o
with	con-, syn-, sym-
within	en-, endo-, intra-
woman	gynec/o
wrist bones	carp/o
x-ray	radi/o

Glossary of English → Spanish Terms*

Here is a list of English → Spanish terms that will help you communicate with Spanish-speaking patients in offices, hospitals, and other medical settings. It includes parts of the body and other medical terms as well.

abdomen	abdomen (ahb-DOH-mehn)
acne	acné (ahk-NEH)
acoustic	acústico (ah-KOOS-tee-ko)
adenoid	adenoide (ah-deh-NOH-ee-deh)
amebic	amébico (ah-MEH-bee-ko)
analgesic	analgésico (ah-nahl-HEH-see-koh)
anemia	anemia (ah-NEH-mee-ah)
anesthesia	anestesia (ah-nehs-TEH-see-ah)
angina	angina (ahn-HEE-na)
angioma	angioma (ahn-hee-OH-mah)
ankle	tobillo (toh-BEE-yoh)
antacid	antiácido (ahn-tee-AH-see-doh)
antiarrhythmic	antiarritmia (ahn-tee-ah-REET-mee-ah)
antibiotic	antibiótico (ahn-tee-bee-OH-tee-koh)
anticonvulsant	anticonvulsivo (ahn-tee-kohn-bool-SEE-boh)
antidiarrheal	antidiarrético (ahn-tee-dee-ah-RHEH-tee-koh)
antiemetic	antiemético (ahn-tee-eh-MEH-tee-koh)
antiepileptic	antiepiléptico (ahn-tee-eh-pee-LEHP-tee-koh)
antihistamine	antihistamínico (ahn-tee-ees-tah-MEE-nee-koh)
antiviral	antivirus (ahn-tee-BEE-roos)
anus	ano (AH-no)
appendix	apéndice (ah-PEHN-dee-seh)
arm	brazo (BRAH-soh)
armpit	axila (ahx-EE-lah)
arteriogram	arteriograma (ahr-teh-ree-oh-GRAH-mah)
arthritis	artritis (ahr-TREE-tees)
asthma	asma (AHS-mah)
bacteria	bacteria (bahk-TEH-ree-ah)
barbiturates	barbitúricos (bahr-bee-TOO-ree-kohs)
birthmark	lunar (loo-NAHR)
bleeding	sangrado (sahn-GRAH-doh)
blood	sangre (SAHN-greh)
blood count	biometría hemática (bee-oh-meh-TREE-ah eh-MAH-tee-kah)
bradycardia	bradicardia (brah-dee-KAHR-dee-ah)
brain	cerebro (seh-REH-bro)
breast/chest	seno (SEH-noh), pecho (PEH-choh)
bronchial tube	bronquio (BROHN-kee-oh)
bronchitis	bronquitis (brohn-KEE-tees)
bruises	moretónes (moh-reh-TOH-nehs)
burn	quemadura (keh-mah-DOO-rah)
buttocks	nalgas (NAHL-gahs)

calf	pantorrilla (pahn-toh-REE-yah)
callus	callo (KAH-yoh)
calm	calma (KAHL-mah)
cardiac	cardiaco (kahr-DEE-ah-koh)
cataract	catarata (kah-tah-RAH-tah)
cervix	cuello uterino (KOO-eh-joh oo-teh-REE-noh), cerviz (SERH-beex)
chancre	chancro (CHAHN-kroh)
cheek	mejilla (meh-HEE-yah)
chemotherapy	quimioterapia (kee-mee-oh-teh-RAH-pee-ah)
chin	barbilla (bar-BEE-ya)
cholesterol	colesterol (koh-lehs-teh-ROHL)
cirrhosis	cirrosis (see-RROH-sees)
claustrophobia	claustrofobia (klah-oos-troh-FOH-bee-ah)
coagulation	coagulación (koh-ah-goo-lah-see-OHN)
collar bone	clavícula (klah-VEE-kuh-la)
colon	colon (KOH-lohn)
constipation	estreñimiento (ehs-treh-nyee-mee-EHN-toh)
cortisone	cortisona (kohr-tee-SOH-nah)
cough	tos (tohs)
cyanotic	cianótico (see-ah-NOH-tee-ko)
decongestants	descongestionantes (dehs-kohn-hehs-tee-oh-NAHN-tehs)
dehydrated	deshidratado (deh-see-drah-TAH-doh)
delirious	delirio (deh-LEE-ree-oh)
depressed	deprimido (deh-pree-MEE-doh)
diabetes	diabetes (dee-ah-BEH-tehs)
diarrhea	diarrea (dee-ah-RREH-ah)
digitalis	digitálicos (dee-hee-TAH-lee-kohs)
ear (inner)	oído (oh-EE-do)
ear (outer)	oreja (oh-REH-hah)
ecchymosis	equimosis (eh-kee-MOH-sees)
eczema	eccema (ehk-SEH-mah)
elbow	codo (KOH-doh)
embolism	embolia (ehm-boh-LEE-ah)
emetic	emético (eh-MEH-tee-koh)
enteritis	enteritis (ehn-teh-REE-tees)
epilepsy	epilepsia (eh-pee-LEHP-see-ah)
euphoric	eufórico (eh-oo-FOH-ree-koh)
exudate	exudado (ehk-soo-DAH-doh)
eye	ojo (OH-hoh)
eyebrow	ceja (SEH-hah)
eyelash	pestaña (pehs-TAH-nyah)
eyelids	párpados (PAHR-pah-dohs)
fibroid	fibroide (fee-BROH-ee-deh)

finger	dedo (DEH-doh)
fingernail	uña (OO-nyah)
fist	puño (POO-nyoh)
fistula	fístula (FEES-too-lah)
foot	pie (pee-EH)
forearm	antebrazo (an-teh-BRAH-zoh)
forehead	frente (FREN-teh)
fungus	hongos (OHN-gohs)

gallbladder	vesícula biliar (beh-SEE-koo-lah bee-lee-AHR)
gangrene	gangrena (gahn-GREH-nah)
gastroenteritis	gastroenteritis (gahs-troh-ehn-teh-REE-tees)
gastroenterology	gastroenterología (gahs-troh-ehn-teh-roh-loh-HEE-ah)
genital organs	órganos genitales (ORH-gah-nohs heh-nee-TAH-lehs)
glaucoma	glaucoma (glah-oo-KOH-mah)
groin	ingle (EEN-gleh)
gums	encías (ehn-SEE-ahs)
gynecologist	ginecólogo (hee-neh-KOH-loh-goh)

hair	cabello (kah-BEH-yoh)
hand	mano (MAH-noh)
head	cabeza (kah-BEH-sah)
heart	corazón (koh-rah-SOHN)
heel	talón (tah-LOHN)
hematology	hematología (eh-mah-toh-loh-HEE-ah)
hematoma	hematoma (eh-mah-TOH-mah)
hemolysis	hemólisis (eh-MOH-lee-sees)
hemorrhage	hemorragia (eh-moh-RRAH-hee-ah)
hepatitis	hepatitis (eh-pah-TEE-tees)
hernia	hernia (EHR-nee-ah)
hip	cadera (kah-DEH-rah)
hypertension	hipertensión (ee-pehr-tehn-see-OHN)

icteric	ictérico (eek-TEH-ree-koh)
infection	infección (een-fehk-see-OHN)
inflammation	inflamación (een-flah-mah-see-OHN)
insulin	insulina (een-soo-LEE-nah)
intestine	intestino (een-tes-TEE-noh)
intramuscular	intramuscular (een-trah-moos-koo-LAHR)
intravenous	intravenoso (een-trah-beh-NOH-soh)
irradiate	irradiar (ee-rrhah-dee-AHR)

jaw	mandíbula (mahn-DEE-boo-lah)

kidney	riñón (ree-NYON)
knee	rodilla (ro-DEE-yah)

laparoscopy	laparoscopía (lah-pah-rohs-KOH-pee-ah)
laryngitis	laringitis (lah-reen-HEE-tees)
laxative	laxante (lahx-AHN-teh)
left	izquierdo (ees-kee-EHR-doh)
leg	pierna (pee-EHR-nah)
ligament	ligamento (lee-gah-MEHN-toh)
lingual	lingual (leen-GUAHL)
lip	labio (LAH-bee-oh)
lithium	litio (LEE-tee-oh)
liver	hígado (EE-gah-doh)
low cholesterol	poco colesterol (POH-koh koh-lehs-teh-ROHL)
low fat	poca grasa (POH-kah GRAH-sah)
low sodium	poca sal (POH-kah sahl)
lung	pulmón (pool-MOHN)
meningitis	meningitis (meh-neen-HEE-tees)
morphine	morfina (mohr-FEE-nah)
mouth	boca (BOH-kah)
muscle	músculo (MOOS-koo-loh)
narcotics	narcóticos (nahr-KOH-tee-kohs)
nasal	nasal (nah-SAHL)
nausea	náusea (NAH-oo-seh-ah)
navel	ombligo (ohm-BLEE-goh)
neck	cuello (koo-EH-yoh)
neonatal	neonatal (neh-oh-nah-TAHL)
nephrologists	nefrólogo (nehp-PHROH-lo-goh)
nephrology	nefrología (neh-phroh-lo-HEEAH)
nervous	nervioso (nehr-bee-OH-soh)
neurotic	neurótico (neh-oo-ROH-tee-koh)
nipple	pezón (peh-SOHN)
nitroglycerin	nitroglicerina (nee-troh-glee-seh-REE-nah)
nose	nariz (nah-REES)
nostrils	fosas nasales (foh-SAHS na-SAH-lehs)
Novocain	novocaina (noh-boh-kah-EE-nah)
nuclear medicine	medicina nuclear (meh-dee-SEE-nah NOO-kleh-ahr)
obstetrics	obstetricia (ohbs-tee-TREE-see-ah)
oncology	oncología (ohn-koh-loh-HEE-ah)
ophthalmic	oftálmico (ohf-TAHL-mee-koh)
ophthalmology	oftalmología (ohf-tahl-moh-loh-HEE-ah)
optic	óptico (OHP-tee-koh)
orthopedics	ortopedia (ohr-toh-PEH-dee-ah)
orthopedic surgeon	cirujano ortopédico (see-roo-HAH-noh ohr-toh-PEH-dee-koh)

otic	ótico (OH-tee-koh)
ovary	ovario (oh-BAH-ree-oh)
palate	paladar (pah-lah-DAHR)
palpation	palpación (pahl-pah-see-OHN)
palpitation	palpitación (pahl-pee-tah-see-OHN)
pancreas	páncreas (PAHN-kreh-ahs)
pancreatitis	pancreatitis (pahn-kreh-ah-TEE-tees)
paralytic	paralítico (pah-rah-LEE-tee-koh)
pathogen	patogen (pah-toh-HEHN)
pathological	patológico (pah-toh-LOH-hee-koh)
pathology	patología (pah-toh-loh-HEE-ah)
pediatrics	pediatría (peh-dee-ah-TREE-ah)
pelvis	pelvis (PEHL-bees)
penis	pene (PEH-neh), miembro (mee-EHM-broh)
pneumonia	pulmonía/neumonía (pool-moh-NEE-ah/neh-oo-moh-NEE-ah)
pruritic	prurito (proo-REE-toh)
psoriasis	soriasis (soh-ree-AH-sees)
psychiatrist	psiquiatra (see-kee-AH-trah)
psychiatry	psiquiatría (see-kee-AH-tree-ah)
psychologist	psicólogo (see-KOH-loh-goh)
pubic	púbico (POO-bee-koh)
pyorrhea	piorrea (pee-oh-RREH-ah)
radiologist	radiólogo (rah-dee-OH-loh-goh)
radiology	radiología (rah-dee-oh-loh-HEEAH)
rectum	recto (REHK-toh)
rheumatic	reumático (reh-oo-MAH-tee-koh)
rib	costilla (kohs-TEE-yah)
right	derecho (deh-REH-choh)
roseola	roseola (roh-seh-OH-lah)
rubella	rubéola (roo-BEH-oh-lah)
scalp	cuero cabelludo (KOO-eh-roh kah-beh-YOO-doh)
sebaceous	sebáceo (seh-BAH-seh-oh)
sedatives	sedativos/sedantes (seh-dah-TEE-bohs/seh-DAHN-tehs)
shin	espinilla (ehs-pee-NEE-yah)
shoulder	hombro (OHM-bro)
skin	piel (pee-EHL)
skull	cráneo (KRAH-ne-oh)
spinal column	columna vertebral (koh-LUHM-nah behr-teh-BRAHL)
spleen	bazo (BAH-zoh), esplín (ehs-PLEEN)
stethoscope	estetoscopio (ehs-teh-tohs-KOH-pee-oh)
stomach	estómago (ehs-TOH-mah-goh)
stool sample	muestra de excremento (moo-EHS-trah deh ehs-kreh-MENH-toh)
straight	derecho (deh-REH-choh)

subaxillary	subaxilar (soob-AHX-ee-lahr)
subcutaneous	subcutáneo (soob-koo-TAH-neh-oh)
sublingual	sublingual (soob-LEEN-goo-ahl)
substernal	substernal (soobs-TEHR-nahl)
surgeon	cirujano (see-roo-HAH-noh)
surgery	cirugía (see-roo-HEE-ah)
symptoms	síntomas (SEEN-toh-mahs)
syncope	síncope (SEEN-koh-peh)
systole	sístole (SEES-toh-leh)
teeth	dientes (dee-EHN-tehs)
temple	sien (see-EHN)
testicles	testículos (tehs-TEE-koo-lohs)
tetanus	tétano (TEH-tah-noh)
therapy	terapia (teh-RAH-pee-ah)
thigh	muslo (MOOS-loh)
throat	garganta (gahr-GAHN-tah)
thyroid	tiroide (tee-ROY-deh)
toes	dedos (DEH-dos), del pié (dehl PEE-eh)
tongue	lengua (LEHN-goo-ah)
tonsillitis	tonsilitis/amigdalitis (tohn-see-LEE-tees/ah-meeg-dah-LEE-tees)
tonsils	amígdalas (ah-MEEG-da-las)
ulcer	úlcera (OOL-seh-rah)
ulnar	ulnar (OOL-nahr)
ultrasound	ultrasonido (ool-trah-soh-NEE-doh)
uremia	uremia (oo-REH-mee-ah)
urinary bladder	vejiga (beh-HEE-gah)
urine	orina (oh-REE-nah)
urticaria	urticaria (oor-tee-KAH-ree-ah)
uterus	útero (OO-teh-roh)
uvula	úvula (OO-boo-lah)
vaginitis	vaginitis (bah-hee-NEE-tees)
vagus	vago (BAH-goh)
valve	válvula (BAHL-boo-lah)
varicocele	varicocele (bah-ree-koh-SEH-leh)
vertigo	vértigo (BEHR-tee-goh)
waist	cintura (sin-TOO-rah)
womb	vientre (bee-EHN-treh)
wrist	muñeca (moo-NYEH-kah)
x-rays	rayos equis (rah-YOHS EH-kees)
zygomatic	cigomático (see-goh-MAH-tee-koh)

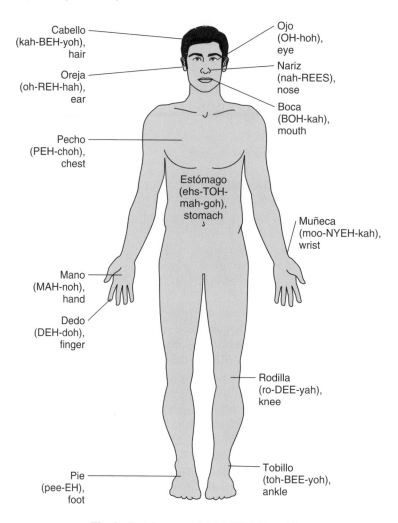

Cabello
(kah-BEH-yoh),
hair

Oreja
(oh-REH-hah),
ear

Pecho
(PEH-choh),
chest

Ojo
(OH-hoh),
eye

Nariz
(nah-REES),
nose

Boca
(BOH-kah),
mouth

Estómago
(ehs-TOH-mah-goh),
stomach

Muñeca
(moo-NYEH-kah),
wrist

Mano
(MAH-noh),
hand

Dedo
(DEH-doh),
finger

Rodilla
(ro-DEE-yah),
knee

Pie
(pee-EH),
foot

Tobillo
(toh-BEE-yoh),
ankle

The body (el cuerpo [ehl-KWEHR-poh]).

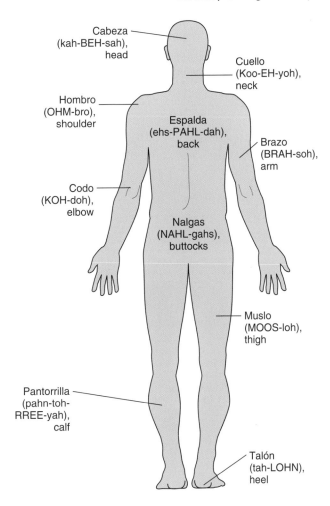

Cabeza
(kah-BEH-sah),
head

Cuello
(Koo-EH-yoh),
neck

Hombro
(OHM-bro),
shoulder

Espalda
(ehs-PAHL-dah),
back

Brazo
(BRAH-soh),
arm

Codo
(KOH-doh),
elbow

Nalgas
(NAHL-gahs),
buttocks

Muslo
(MOOS-loh),
thigh

Pantorrilla
(pahn-toh-
RREE-yah),
calf

Talón
(tah-LOHN),
heel

The body (el cuerpo [ehl-KWEHR-poh]).

Index

Page numbers followed by f indicate figures; t, tables.

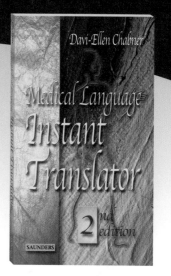